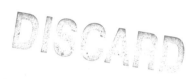

The Newly Qualified Nurse's Handbook

A SURVIVAL GUIDE

Commissioning Editor: Ninette Premdas
Development Editor: Sheila Black
Project Manager: Elouise Ball
Design Manager: George Ajayi

The Newly Qualified Nurse's Handbook

A SURVIVAL GUIDE

Bethann Siviter RN (Adult) BSc (Hons) Dip (HE) SPDN
Consultant Nurse
Past Chair of the RCN Association of Nursing Students

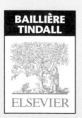

BAILLIÈRE
TINDALL

ELSEVIER

Edinburgh   London   New York   Oxford
Philadelphia   St Louis   Sydney   Toronto   2008

BAILLIÈRE
TINDALL
ELSEVIER

An imprint of Elsevier Limited

First published 2008

978-0-7020-2803-8

British Library Cataloguing in Publication Data
A catalogue record for this book is available from the British Library

Library of Congress Cataloging in Publication Data
A catalog record for this book is available from the Library of Congress

Notice
Neither the Publisher nor the Author assumes any responsibility for any loss or injury and/or damage to persons or property arising out of or related to any use of the material contained in this book. It is the responsibility of the treating practitioner, relying on independent expertise and knowledge of the patient, to determine the best treatment and method of application for the patient.

The Publisher

ELSEVIER | your source for books, journals and multimedia in the health sciences
www.elsevierhealth.com

The publisher's policy is to use paper manufactured from sustainable forests

Printed in China

Contents

Foreword

I knew when I read Bethan Siviter's first book *The Student Nurse's Handbook* that this book, *The Newly Qualified Nurse's Handbook* just had to be written. Here it is. And it is everything I could have hoped for – and more!

Many people believe (wrongly) that nursing is just about doing tasks and procedures, and might expect this *Handbook* to be a bit like a procedure manual, with instructions and tips about complicated techniques for things like dressing wounds or managing intravenous infusions. There are other books on the market that fulfil that role.

But that is not what nursing is about and it is not what this *Handbook* is about. Nursing practice is about making difficult decisions in complex situations. It is more about managing people (including one's professional self) than dealing with complicated equipment. The trouble is that few pre-registration programmes prepare nurses for this reality and there are very few books about it.

That's exactly where *The Newly Qualified Nurse's Handbook* comes in. Here is everything that the newly qualified nurse wants and needs to know but was afraid to ask. On the one hand, it is scholarly – extremely well researched and evidence based. But it is also intensely practical, filled with real-life scenarios and suggestions, based on a deep understanding of nursing and how it feels to be a nurse. And best of all (given that nursing is a tough job and a little humour helps lighten the load), it is fun to read.

I just wish it had been around when I was a newly qualified nurse!

Professor Dame June Clark DBE PhD RN FRCN
Professor Emeritus, Swansea University

Preface

First, just a reminder: for ease of reading (and writing) I will usually say 'patients' when I refer to those for whom nurses care and usually refer to nurses as female. This isn't intended to stereotype anyone and does not imply any lack of respect, prejudice or bias.

I want to thank all of you who read *The student nurse handbook* and who have encouraged me to write more. I also want to thank all of you who encouraged me to write this book. But let me tell you why it took so long to get here.

In 2005, I fell seriously ill and wound up, for a good part of 2006, being not a nurse but a patient. I spent countless weeks in hospital and then receiving home care support, on consultant waiting lists, sitting in offices for professionals from nurses to physios to even more doctors . . . and I realised that this book, which was nearing completion, needed to be something more.

When it was first written, it was written as a nurse to a nurse. But, as a patient, I realised that many of the nurses had no idea how I was feeling. There were a number of dedicated, caring, intuitive and very skilled nurses who helped me tremendously. There were also a fair number of nurses – many of them new to the profession – who harmed me, not intentionally, through their lack of awareness, lack of skill and lack of attention to detail and follow-through. Despite my own physical pain, I was even more hurt by the pain of seeing this profession, which I love, in tatters and turmoil.

I realised, in this pain, that I needed to give something more than just a guide from a nurse to a nurse – I realised that what you and nurses like you needed and wanted was insight on how to take good care of patients so that they would get better, despite the overwhelming responsibilities, conflicting demands and time constraints you face every day, despite staffing problems and cuts, and still know that you had done the best possible to help them.

I met a fair many bad nurses who caused me much harm and heartache; a few were intentionally uncaring but more often they were well-meaning people who, rushed off their feet, neglected simple but important things. There were some excellent HCAs and my spirits were buoyed by the students who, recognising my name, wanted to talk to me.

The bad nurses I encountered drove me to both fear and dread my encounters with them. They were haphazard, forgot things, left things undone, spoke ill of their patients within earshot of others, failed to assess appropriately, failed to do what was ordered and failed to care. They thought giving medication on time was enough to be a nurse.

But, back to the good nurses – what they shared was consistent: they were attentive, honest, patient and forgiving. They came back when they said they would, they assessed me and followed-through when there was a problem, and they held my hand and let me cry when there was nothing else to do. They didn't wait for me to ask – they knew what I needed and made sure my needs were met. They kept me fed, watered, clean and as comfortable as possible even when I was cranky, miserable and didn't trust them as far as I could throw them, and considering that I couldn't even stand that wasn't very far!

You know what happened as a result of the failings of the other nurses? I became angry, withdrawn, and completely distrustful of the nursing staff. You have all had patients like me: the ones everyone hates to go in to because you get nothing back from them; the patient who says 'Like you would anyway!' when you ask if there is anything you can do to make them more comfortable.

What I will ask, on behalf of those patients, is that you persevere. They are afraid; they have been taught that no matter how much they ask for help, no-one will help them; they are paralysed by pain that has no relief and unrelenting fear of what is happening to their bodies . . . sit by them, hold their hand, no matter what they say – and for heaven's sake, do what you say you will do. When you can turn one of those patients around, get them to trust and have faith in nurses again, as the loving and caring sister of A1 did for me (my gratitude knows no bounds to that one nurse), then you will really be the kind of nurse you need to be.

This is the kind of nurse you need to be: don't wait for patients to ask – meet their needs in advance. Don't make them wait for care they need. Don't make them beg. Don't leave them in pain. Don't make things worse for them. Respect them as people, even the ones who are lost in a fog of dementia or confusion or who have lost their ability to move, communicate, care for themselves . . . Care for them all as if they were family, love them, and love the unlovable ones even more!

I hope I can always be that kind of nurse, and I hope you will be that kind of nurse too, because that is the kind of nurse the patient today needs us to be.

On your journey in this wonderful profession, I offer you my praise, my support and also my sympathy. It's a hard road, but I can't imagine a better one.

Oh, I nearly forgot: I need to thank one other group, although they will likely never read this. Thank you, to the other patients who shared a ward with me – we did take care of each other girls, didn't we? Thanks for teaching me so much about being a nurse and I hope I can always strive be the nurse that you and others like you need me to be.

Bethann Siviter
Birmingham, 2008

Acknowledgements

As always, I need to thank my husband, Andrew, for being my friend and partner and for being the constant and unyielding support for everything I do in life. I need to acknowledge my Mum, a recently retired cardiac nurse, who taught me so much about the spirit and art of nursing, and my Dad, 'CioCia' Rita and Uncle John for teaching me the value of unconditional love and acceptance. I need to thank my friend Jane Gardiner for being not only a true friend but a caring and skilled nurse when I needed her to be one, Lynne Young and my dear friend Gill Robertson from the RCN, Les Storey for being such an able and willing teacher with such a useful brutally honest streak, my friend Theresa Clarke. Very sincere and heartfelt thanks to Professor John Raphael, Sister Jane Southall and the incredible Rheumatology Nurses at Russell's Hall Hospital for giving me back a life worth living – I know I am the world's worst patient, but thank you for seeing through the fear and anxiety and treating me with such compassion and patience; and of course also Elsevier and my poor beleaguered but patient editor Ninette Premdas for persevering with me when it seemed hopeless.

To:

Andrew Siviter
John and Regina Stavaski
William and Dorothy Vaitkunas

and to my patients:

thank you for allowing me the privilege of being your nurse

1 Working as a nurse

- Transition from student to staff nurse
- Power and hierarchies in nursing
- Choosing your work environment
- Being the nurse you want to be
- Direct entry into community nursing
- Specialist and advanced practice
- Boards and committees
- Post-qualification education
- Summary
- Poem: *See me*

"As a first year student I felt like it was never going to end. It was the longest year of my life. Second year was tough, and by the end I felt like quitting. I was so burned out and frustrated. A couple of third years said it was like that for them too, and that it would get better. It did – the third year flew. I was waiting for my PIN in no time. Then the real panic started! (newly qualified nurse)"

TRANSITION FROM STUDENT TO STAFF NURSE

It might seem as though the transition from student to staff nurse starts as soon as you get your PIN; in reality it starts from the moment you started your course. Every day, every step you took, was bringing you closer to being a nurse. In fact, some of the things you probably took for granted as a student were excellent preparation for starting your new nursing role. Think about this – how many times did you have to learn:

- where everything was
- the way things were documented
- everyone's name and face
- the network of departments and telephone numbers
- about shifts and the off duty.

Many people starting a new job say that these are the kinds of things that are most frustrating. As a new nurse (and very experienced student) you have had a lot of experience being 'new'. You have developed excellent coping skills to help you adapt quickly to the environment in which you will be working – you might not realise how well prepared you are.

Most new nurses have worries. To show you how well prepared you really are, let's take a look at some of those worries one by one.

'I really don't know what I am doing . . .'

You're partly right. There are many things you don't know. But what are you really expecting from yourself? Are you expecting to have all the answers and to be as knowledgeable and skilled as a senior nurse with years of experience? And what are other people expecting of you? The truth is that other staff members are expecting you to:

- Know how to behave in a professional manner (wear the right uniform, be on time, etc.).
- Know the legal and ethical principles underpinning practice.
- Know how to communicate appropriately.
- Know how to work as a team member.
- Know how to ask for help.

As far as skills, they are expecting that you will:

- Be competent in giving the basic, fundamental care appropriate for your practice area.
- Give medications competently.
- Be able to delegate basic tasks to others in the team.
- Complete a basic assessment competently.
- Know enough to ask for help and support in doing those things you are not yet confident or competent enough to do on your own.

Is there anything in these two lists that wasn't there for you as a final year student? The only real difference is that instead of someone else chasing you to make sure you are doing everything you should, you will be responsible for making sure on your own, with support from a preceptor and from other staff members. As a newly qualified nurse, the only thing that has really changed is your *accountability*. The expectation for your level of skill and knowledge is virtually the same as when you were a final-year student.

'What if I kill someone? Or make a really bad mistake? I don't want to lose my PIN!'

Have you killed anyone yet? No? Good. Not surprising, really, that you haven't – mistakes are usually the result of bad or careless practice. If you want to take the best care of your patients, remember that you should never, ever, act beyond the scope of your knowledge and skill.

There is nothing wrong, even as an experienced qualified nurse, in going to someone and saying 'I need help'.

If you remember nothing else from this entire book, remember that it's always better to ask for help than to forge forward and try to do something you aren't prepared or experienced enough to do.

The truth is, though, that four common problems can 'help' you make mistakes. Avoiding these will help you not make mistakes. Avoid:

1. Being cocky: trying to pretend you are more experienced and skilled than you really are.
2. Being careless: not giving full attention to what you are doing.
3. Being burned out: being so tired, stressed or distracted that you can't keep track of what you are doing.
4. Being disorganised: not having a good grasp on what you need to do and when you need to do it.

You know that you have to pay attention to what you are doing if you are going to avoid mistakes. That means having a plan for what you need to do, not getting flustered or stressed, taking care of yourself, knowing your limits and not taking short cuts. Later on in the book I'll be helping you to plan and to avoid stress. For now, though, just accept that during your nursing career you will make mistakes. Most of them will be small mistakes; a few will be big ones. If you do make a mistake, remember these simple rules:

- **Always own up to a mistake as soon as you realise you have made it:** being honest is essential: you will get into far more trouble if someone else finds out you've made a mistake and you haven't owned up to it. Most importantly, be honest about the reason(s) the mistake was made: don't blame anyone else if it was really your fault.
- **Reflect and learn from your mistakes:** the worst thing you can do with a mistake is to try to pretend that it never happened. Look back, honestly, and see what happened. Then you can make sure it doesn't happen again.
- **Don't let the mistake haunt you:** once it's over, you've reflected on it and learned from it, it's time to let it go. You won't do yourself, your colleagues or your patients any good by dwelling on mistakes.
- **Whatever you do, make sure you put the patient first:** don't get so worried about a mistake that you forget to take care of the patient involved. If you get so upset that you can't think straight, get someone else to help you.

As far as losing your PIN goes, the Nursing and Midwifery Council (NMC) isn't there to be the big bad wolf – it's there to protect the public and to support nurses. You will lose your PIN only if the NMC feels that your practice is so unsafe that the only way to protect the public is for you not to be a nurse. Also, most mistakes aren't anywhere near the level that would need to be referred to the NMC. Issues that *do* go to the NMC show such a shocking lack of skill, knowledge or judgement that the nurse simply can't be allowed to continue. Statistically, nurses with many years of experience are more likely to be called before the NMC than newly qualified nurses. Why? Because they let their standards slip, got careless, didn't keep up to date or started to take the basic, fundamental nursing principles for granted. If you keep yourself up to date, reflect regularly and make sure you are always doing the right things for the right reasons, you won't have anything to worry about.

If you are ever worried about a decision you have to make or about circumstances at your place of work, you can call the NMC advice line. The people you talk to are knowledgeable, and will give you good, confidential advice. There is more about the NMC, including contact details, in Chapter 9.

'I'm going back to where I worked before, what if they don't accept me as a nurse?' or 'I'm so new – what if they don't accept me?'

It's up to you to be comfortable in your role; if you are comfortable, other people will be comfortable too. Some things might be difficult; for example, asking a healthcare assistant (HCA) to do something for you when that person used to be senior to you when you were training. Here are a few of tips to help you:

- **Be respectful of everyone, regardless of his or her role:** you are no better than any other team member because you are a nurse: sometimes people might be afraid that you will be 'above' them now that you are qualified, and that will cause problems for your team. Be willing to learn from every team member.
- **Don't skive:** delegate appropriately; don't ask someone else to do something for you just because you can (more on delegation in Chapter 3).
- **Don't try *not* to be a nurse:** don't try to fit in by being an HCA. You owe it to the other staff and to the patients to be a nurse. Although it might win a few people over if you take the heaviest assignment, if it takes you away from the things that only a nurse can do, then it will cause you problems.
- **Ask for help if you need it:** don't be worried that if you ask for help people will think you aren't competent: people who don't ask for

help make more experienced staff worry because experienced nurses *know* that, as a newly qualified nurse, you will need help. If you aren't asking for help, then those staff will worry that you are unsafe.

As you can see, you already have the basics you need to be a competent new nurse: all of the expectations – that you would ask for help if you needed it, that you would reflect on your actions and practice, that you would work as a member of a team, and that you would treat others with respect – are things you already know and have been assessed on while a student.

The transition from student to staff nurse is frightening but it really is only one step *in the middle* of a long progression of steps leading to really being a nurse.

Let me give you an example from my own practice. When I was appointed to a senior nursing role, the first things I thought about were:

- What if I make a mistake?
- What if I don't really know what I am doing as well as I should?
- What if they don't accept me?

Does that sound familiar? This is because the steps you take come in two kinds: the little day-to-day steps that you won't notice and the big landmark steps like getting your PIN or changing to a more senior job. You will have the same fears and worries about *every* landmark step as you have about the step between being a student and being a qualified nurse.

Because you don't notice the day-to-day steps, you don't really see how far you have come and how much you have grown. This is where reflection is so important. In my case, I went to another person (my friend Linda) who was in a similar role as my new job and asked how she had felt. I had reflected at length about my skills, my knowledge and my experiences; I shared these reflections with Linda. To my great surprise, when she started her new role years before she had felt same as I was feeling. That's when I realised that it wasn't me – it was the nature of changing roles.

By reflecting, I could answer my doubts about my skills and experience. I could say 'OK, you might be worried, but you *do* have the basics you need to take on this new role.' And you can say that too. If you were a competent and safe final-year student, you *are* a competent and safe newly qualified nurse. Don't let your doubts and fears distract you from the joy and personal growth that awaits you in your new career.

POWER AND HIERARCHIES IN NURSING

The structure of the nursing profession is based on that of the military, probably because the first nursing hierarchies developed in the context of military hospitals and wars. Let's look at all the roles:

> Cadet nurse – Auxiliary nurse – First-year student – Final-year student – Newly qualified nurse –Junior staff nurse – Staff nurse – Senior staff nurse – Junior sister/Charge nurse – Sister/Charge nurse –Senior sister/Charge nurse – Deputy assistant ward manager – Assistant ward manager – Ward manager – Deputy matron – Matron – Clinical nurse – Specialist nurse practitioner – Advanced nurse practitioner – Nurse consultant – Nurse Professor – and should there be Doctor of nursing?

Through all these titles, there is a hierarchy.

An old joke about snobbery and social hierarchies in Boston – the part of America I come from – goes like this:

> I live in Boston town, where the folks are a wee bit odd . . .
> for the Lowells only talk to the Cabots . . .
> and the Cabots only to God.

In the old days, cadets spoke only to student nurses, student nurses to staff nurses, staff nurses to Matron, and Matron to whomever she wished. It's different now, but some patients don't know that. They – especially older ones – might feel the need to ask permission to speak to someone.

'Next to the patient, the most important person in healthcare is next to the patient . . .'

Everyone – from Doctor to Consultant to Sister to Domestic to Student – is worthy of respect and should expect to be treated with the same dignity and be appreciated for their worthiness. In my opinion, the most important nurse is the one who spends the most time with patients giving direct care – and that's most often the HCA: the one there giving care is most important.

Gossiping, back biting, giving junior staff or students the worst assignments – these are all ways of perpetuating a system of fear and intimidation. Everyone should have the same chance to not work Christmas as anyone else. Everyone should believe that their team will support them even if they don't have a degree or a qualification.

Some nurses say they don't get along with physiotherapists or occupational therapists, or they say it's not right that physios don't respect the nurses''authority' on the ward. I heard one sister say: 'That physio prances in and takes patients before we have had a chance to finish with them!' Naughty physio – nicking patients before they're all used up. Seriously though, these things cause real problems.

If you communicate well, treat everyone with respect and learn about what others in your area do, you will avoid the conflicts and hierarchies that drive everyone mad. Trust me, it's either that or always feeling as though you are on the outside. Even doctors today are willing to speak to nurses, or so I've been told!

In fact, doctors have a lot to teach nurses. Most people really want an easy life – at home, at work, everywhere. If your area has a regular doctor, or if you are in a GP's surgery, take the time to find out how the doctor likes things. You are not being the GP's hand-maiden, you are being a team member, and that's a worthy role. By making things better for members of other disciplines, you make them better for your patients and that's really what it's all about.

Working collaboratively as part of a multidisciplinary team is a sure way of promoting nursing as a key, integral profession: not one that is superior to others but also not one that is worth any less than any of them.

How well you work collaboratively will influence the care your patients receive: the better you communicate and work with thera-pists, the better your patients' therapy will be; the better you work with the medics, the better your patients' medical care will be. Is there any better incentive to work collaboratively, share information and under-stand what others need to know than to see your patients getting better care from you by getting better care from others?

CHOOSING YOUR WORK ENVIRONMENT

As a nurse, you will have many different options and opportunities. Some of them might seem very appealing – until you actually start working there and you find that it's not what you really wanted. Knowing this, many Trusts have 'rotation' programmes to allow new nurses to spend time in a number of different areas over their first 1–2 years. It's like having a buffet of opportunities; after you have a taste of each, you might have a better idea what you want for your 'main meal'.

Sometimes, you have to spend time in one job to get into another. An example of this is health visiting; being a health visitor requires a specialist qualification, so you have to work in another post while you work on gaining the experience you need to train as a health visitor.

This tells you something important: if you don't know where you are going, you won't know how to get there. We will discuss continuous professional development (CPD) in Chapter 10. You should plan your CPD to help you advance in your career. But what if you don't know what you really want to do? There are some basic things to think about:

- Can I be flexible or do I need a job that is more stable in hours?
- Can I work full time or do I need part time work?
- Is there something that really interests me? Or something that really puts me off?
- Are there some things I might find emotionally very difficult? Or very rewarding?
- Are there some things that might pose more of a risk than I can accept?
- Are there some things that I already have some experience in?
- What kind of a person am I? Do I like a slow, steady pace? Do I like working alone? Do I thrive on adrenaline? Do I get stressed if I have too many things to do at once?
- Where do I want my career to go?

If you think of these things, it can give you some direction. Let's take Kumar as an example.

Kumar is a newly qualifying mental health nurse. He has been thinking about where to work – the professional journals are full of opportunities for mental health nurses. He makes a shopping list of things he wants from his work, and what he can offer:

- I like being around people all day; I don't like to work alone.
- I like being able to see the people I work with make changes and get better; I think I would struggle with being in a long-term care situation.
- I think I would like to work with people from Asian cultures because I feel there is a gap in available services.
- I don't mind being on call occasionally.
- I can manage a number of different priorities at one time.
- I would like to eventually be involved in developing nurse-led services.

Kumar looks at a few of the jobs on offer in a nursing journal:

1. Forensic mental health unit.
2. Community mental health nurse.
3. Numerous opportunities for nurses at a psychiatric hospital.
4. Children's/young people's services in a Health Trust 25 miles away.
5. Outreach worker in a service for domestic violence.

For each of these, Kumar weighs what they offer against his list. He decides not to apply for the community mental health post because he doesn't feel he would enjoy all the time on his own. He might consider forensics, so he puts that ad to one side. He doesn't want to work in long-term care, so he disregards the hospital posts. He likes children but the job is too far away.

When he reads the ad for the outreach worker, he finds that it 'feels' right. *'Work with women and families from the Asian Community . . .', 'Busy outreach centre', 'Nurse-led services . . .'.* He decides to apply for both the position in the forensic unit and for the outreach worker post.

Because Kumar has some idea of his likes and dislikes, he had a better idea what kinds of opportunities would interest him.

Gill has a different kind of problem in choosing what kind of job to look for.

Before becoming a learning disability nurse, Gill worked as a home manager for 7 years. She feels very confident about her skills in both nursing and management as a result. Originally, she thought she should apply only for entry-level nursing posts but she has realised she might struggle in a post where the manager was weak. Knowing this, she has applied for a post of team leader. In the interview, she outlined the skills and experience she gained from her years in home management, and how she integrated that knowledge into her nursing. Gill was able to show that she was not the same as a new nurse who didn't have the high level of experience she had.

Both these examples show that:

- You have to think about what you want from your career.
- You have to know your strengths and weaknesses.
- You should remember about your 'life before nursing' (LBN) and not discount the valuable experience and knowledge it has given you.
- Just because you are newly qualified doesn't necessarily mean you don't have choices and options.

Your career is yours and you should look for the opportunities that allow you to be the nurse you really want to be.

Remember that the *Improving working lives* document (published by the Department of Health in 2001), and similar initiatives, oblige employers to help you meet family obligations. You should be able to discuss and negotiate flexible working arrangements, shift patterns and shift times that allow you to manage childcare (or other caring) commitments. It is not always possible to have all the accommodations you need but it is getting easier to have a family life and a good career as a nurse. If you have special family obligations, ask about how *Improving working lives* might help.

Working abroad

One option you might consider is working abroad. You should consider a number of factors:

- Are your qualifications transferable or will you need to take extra courses, exams, etc.?
- Are the work patterns different in the country you are considering?
- What language(s) will you need to speak?
- How do nursing and health care differ in the country you are considering?
- Where will you live? Will you be able to drive or will you need a new licence?
- Will you need a work permit?
- How much will it cost to call/visit home?

If you are planning to work abroad, you will probably go through an agency. Agencies that recruit for overseas employers offer considerable help and support to applicants. However, it is not always as clear as it seems:

- Some agencies will charge you a substantial fee if you don't complete an assignment.
- Some agencies provide tickets and travel, some don't.
- Some agencies will help you get necessary exams/courses, some won't.
- Sometimes, you might be promised a particular work environment or living accommodation but have to wait for it to be sorted out after you have arrived in the new country.

As a person who moved from one country to another, I can tell you there are some other things that people might not always think about:

- Nursing is different in different countries: how will you cope and adapt with different practices, laws and professional expectations and still be a safe, competent practitioner?

- Even between countries that speak English there are language differences: are you ready to cope with not spelling or pronouncing
something properly? Or not knowing the right word?
- Have you ever been away from home for a year – so far away that
it took a long flight to get back?
- How do your friends and family feel about it?
- Will you need health insurance and how much will it cost?
- Are there social norms or laws you need to understand: drinking,
smoking, what to wear in public, etc.?

Another option for working abroad is through a voluntary agency or
charity. There are opportunities to work all over the world, with some
very needy people. Assignments vary from a few weeks to a few
months and are sometimes in places where there is ongoing conflict.
You can contact organisations such as:

- The British Red Cross: 44 Moorfields, London EC2Y 9AL. Tel: 0870
170 7000; fax: 020 7562 2000; web address: http://www.redcross.
org.uk
- Médecins Sans Frontières (MSF UK): 67–74 Saffron Hill, London
EC1N 8QX. Tel: 020 7404 6600; fax: 020 7404 4466; web address:
http://www.msf.org/unitedkingdom/

Another way of working abroad is through the military (there is more
on this in the next section).

Working abroad is a wonderful opportunity but it is something you
need to consider carefully. Just because it's nice to visit somewhere
doesn't mean it will be that exciting to work there. Make certain that
any promises an agency makes are in writing and that you won't be
penalised for backing out if the agency doesn't keep its promises. If
you are seriously thinking of going abroad, contact your union or
professional organisation for advice.

Working in the military

The Territorial Army (TA) Medical Service is one option if you want to
work in the military, or you might want to be a nurse in the Army or
Royal Navy. There are excellent opportunities for nurses, in very varied
settings and environments. Depending on where you want to go with
your career, the military could give you an exceptional foundation.
Some benefits of being a military nurse are:

- opportunities to really improve your physical fitness
- confidence building
- financial benefits
- training, skills and knowledge
- varied opportunities in many different areas and settings.

You can contact the TA for more information, the web address is: http://www.ta.mod.uk or ring 0845 603 8000. The postal and regular contacts all vary by area, so you need to look up your local contact.

If you are interested in being in the Army or Royal Navy, you should contact a local recruiting office or look at http://www.mod.uk.

Working 'on the bank'/working agency

Some people find working 'on the bank' or working for an agency to be a lucrative and flexible option to working regular shifts. As a former nursing student, you know about working bank shifts!

The bank

Many Trusts or organisations will have their own staff bank. Staff register and then pick the shifts they would like to work from the available open shifts. Sometimes, a staff member might even be called and asked to work an open shift at the last minute. Working the bank can often mean greater flexibility and a higher wage than that usually paid. It does not, however, count towards regular hours or towards overtime. The NHS has its own 'bank': NHS Professionals.

Agency

There are many different nurse staffing agencies. They all have different incentives and benefits, and different pay.

- Pros: flexible hours and shifts, you don't have to work in places you don't like, the pay is good.
- Cons: unpredictable working patterns, inconsistent income, you might be moved from the area you booked to another one, shifts are sometimes cancelled at last minute.

As a nurse, you also have professional considerations:

- You must be certain that you are able to safely and competently deliver nursing care. What if you are inexperienced and you are the only nurse?
- You must be able to work with staff that you might not know very well. Are you able to delegate things without knowing the person? What would you need to know to be confident about delegating?
- You shouldn't work so many hours that you become stressed, overly fatigued or distracted.

Working 'bank' or agency can be an excellent opportunity but, as a nurse, you have a higher level of accountability and responsibility. If you are working in unfamiliar areas you might need a lot of confidence! Make sure when you are booking shifts that you will have the support you need.

BEING THE NURSE YOU WANT TO BE

Do you remember when you first decided to become a nurse? You had an image in your head of the kind of person a nurse was. What were the qualities you thought a nurse should have? How did a nurse behave? Who did you see yourself becoming?

Think back to the last shift you worked. How different is 'real life' from what you thought it would be? Some of the qualities often attributed to nurses are very appropriate:

● patient
● kind
● caring
● genuine
● honest
● knowledgeable
● skilled.

Some are not appropriate:

● self-sacrificing
● the demanding matron
● domineering
● 'nurse knows best'.

The reality is that you won't become the nurse you thought you were going to be because you didn't know a lot about nursing when you first got the image in your mind. Now that you have been through nurse education, you know the real qualities in a nurse:

Think about who you would be if you were really able to be the nurse you want to be. Get an image from the positive role models you have encountered. Think of the things you saw nurses (and other professionals) do that impressed you. Now, think of the more negative role models – what did they do that you promised yourself you would never do?

If you're anything like most people, these are a few of the things you said about bad practice:

● 'I'm *never* going to do manual handling that way! I'll always do it the right way!'
● 'I'm *never* going to treat a student the way I was treated'
● 'I'm *never* going to be too busy for *my* patients'.

But it's likely that even by the time you finished your course you had already started to slip. In Chapter 6 we will talk about reflection (oh stop groaning, it's not that bad!) but for now I would like you just to think about the areas you have started to slip.

Are you the nurse you wanted to be *right now*? I'm not referring to experience – that will come with time – I'm talking about the way you think and what your priorities are. Right now, I would like to challenge you to accept a mission: always put the patient first. This doesn't mean doing things you shouldn't do – such as washing someone who should wash themselves or being foolish by giving up all your breaks and working unpaid overtime – it means making sure that all your decisions, about everything you do, are based on the patient's best interest. Thinking back, the nurse you wanted to be was one who did exactly that – always put the patient first.

Periodically, think about the nurse you are becoming. Look around you for the good role models and the people who are supporting you. Look at the negative role models – keep those promises you made to yourself – 'I'm *never* . . .' – don't develop amnesia!

Becoming the nurse you want to be . . . it's really very easy: just work hard not to become the nurse you *don't* want to be!

DIRECT ENTRY INTO COMMUNITY NURSING

For many nurses, the biggest myth about community nursing is that you can't work in the community until you have had 'X' years' experience in the hospital. The truth is that as primary care expands to meet more needs in the community there are many entry-level opportunities for nurses to start their career in the community.

Although the professional skills depend on your branch, the following is a general skill set essential for community working:

- a current driving licence
- confidence
- being self directed
- being well organised
- being adaptable and flexible
- having excellent communication skills
- having good documentation skills
- being a good decision maker
- having good evidence-based practice
- being able to manage interruptions and unpredictable events.

In the community, you will often find that you are working on your own. You will receive direction from your manager or senior nurse but, when you are with a patient, there might not be anyone else there with you. This varies with the setting, but to work successfully in the community you have to have a sense of responsibility for managing your own workload.

If you are in adult or children's nursing and want to work in the community, it would help to foster the skills you would need:

- wound care (theory and products)
- strong assessment skills (including spirometry, use of a Doppler, etc.)
- knowledge of long-term and chronic conditions and the relevant nursing skills
- phlebotomy
- use of equipment: manual handling equipment, adaptive equipment, etc.
- critical decision making.

This isn't to say that you have to be able to do a Doppler examination before you can apply to be a community nurse, but it will help you when you apply if you at least know what a Doppler is and what kind of information it gives the nurse (just so you know, a Doppler is used to determine if someone has venous or arterial disease in their legs; it helps the nurse determine if it is safe to put the patient in compression bandages).

In mental health and learning disability nursing there are fewer barriers to working in the community because each of these areas has strong community service networks. You might find that you are not working on your own so much in these areas, and that there are opportunities for jobs in very diverse areas.

Here is the pathway one nurse, Jane Gardiner, took to develop her career in the community. Jane is now a qualified District Nurse. As she approached her qualification as a nurse in 2002, she planned ahead because she wanted to work in the community:

I knew community was where I wanted to work, so I set myself goals, starting in my final year as a student. My goals were:

1. Get the foundation I need to be a community nurse when I qualify.
2. Make the connections I need so when I go to apply I can get good advice and support.

When I qualified, because I had met my first two goals, I was able to get a community nurse post. I then set more goals:

1. To be an E grade in 12 months.
2. To become a district nurse within 3 years.
3. To develop a very strong skill set in wound care within 1 year.

As a third-year student, I took every relevant in-service and training my placement area would let me take. I looked for opportunities to gain the kinds of knowledge and skill that community nurses should have. Some of the courses were:

● wound care
● continence assessment
● medications and drugs in the community
● feeding tubes
● stoma care.

I also spent time with specialist nurses like tracheostomy nurses, diabetes nurses and MacMillan nurses. As I arranged my placements, I looked for areas that I could connect to nursing in the community. I also spoke with my mentor on my community placement: she gave me advice and guidance about how I should prepare to be a community nurse. Our Trust even put on sessions to help us prepare to be community nurses!

One of the sessions told us what kinds of things to put on our application, which fell into the following areas:

● Why we wanted to be community nurses.
● The special qualities community nurses have.
● What the difference was between working in the community and working in the hospital.
● What the patients/their families/carers should expect from a community nurse.

Looking back at those questions now, I realise that I did have a good idea about what community nursing would be. I felt that nursing really began in the community – it is where most of the people are most of the time, healthy, sick, in between!

For 8 months I worked as a D grade nurse; during that time, my manager and I were working on a programme to help me develop the skills I needed to move to E grade. I needed to be able to do ear syringing, develop more advanced wound care, go on a mentor's course and meet the Trust guidelines for the more advanced role. I had to show that I was moving from the basic skills to the more advanced skills.

As an E grade I started to support students and some of the healthcare assistants. I started to develop more time-management skills and to look at the team's work, not just my own. After a while, I realised that I was ready for the district nursing course. I started feeling like I should be doing more, and that my nursing was at a level where I was ready to take on more responsibility. In fact, I had already started to take on some additional responsibilities at a higher level. I felt that I was starting to think at a higher level and I could do more as a specialist community nurse. I spoke with my district nurse and she really encouraged me. The management in my Trust also was very supportive. The course was stressful but it has changed me as a person and a nurse, and I am looking forward to setting some new goals for this next stage of my career, as a district nurse!

One thing I always want to remember: as a nurse, in whatever capacity I work, I always want to be the nurse my patient needs me to be. This was brought home for me by the poem *Who do you see when you are looking at me?* [this appears at the end of this chapter]. It was given me during my preparation as a district nurse, and I feel every nurse should read it.

Jane's story shows how one nurse planned ahead and made the move directly into community nursing. Looking back at her story, we see:

- She had a definite plan.
- The plan included preparing to meet the basic requirements for the job she wanted.
- She kept planning as she reached the different stages of her development.
- She accepted help from other people.
- She grew in knowledge, skill and confidence.

If you really want to work in the community, there will be a job for you – if you are prepared to show how you are the right nurse for the job.

SPECIALIST AND ADVANCED PRACTICE

A specialist knows more about a particular area than anyone else. Specialists can practise in specific clinical areas (like diabetes or wound care) or work in a general area (such as in the care of older people).

They often give advice to other providers in addition to providing care themselves.

Most specialists gain their knowledge through a combination of work experience and education. If you find that you are really attracted to one certain area of practice, it might be worthwhile to find someone who is a specialist and ask what the job entails, and what qualifications and experience are needed to do the job. Most specialist roles require a degree or evidence of degree-level preparation for the role.

Like specialist practice, advanced practice is a mixed bag of experience and education, and can be in general or specific clinical areas. The hallmarks of what most people would refer to as 'advanced practice' also apply to specialist roles:

- **Expert clinical skills in an area of nursing:** feeling confident and comfortable as a practitioner, and having a wide experience base.
- **Ability to research and use evidence to determine practice:** being able both to understand and to do research and audit (see Chapter 4 for more information on research and evidence-based practice).
- **Leadership skills** (see Chapter 5 for more information on leadership).
- **Recognised by peers as a clinical leader:** advanced practitioners exhibit 'influence' – other staff will seek their advice.
- **Critical thinking and reasoning** (see Chapter 4 for more information on critical thinking).
- **Intuition:** somehow, advanced nurses seem to 'know' things (see Chapter 6 for more on intuition).
- **Autonomy:** the ability and authority to act independently.
- **Teaching, mentorship:** the knowledge, skill and desire to teach and support the development of colleagues and students (there is more in Chapter 7 about mentorship).

In general, advanced and specialist practitioners are leaders in improving care and nursing practice. These nurses are role models not just for other nurses but across the multidisciplinary team.

These advanced nurses don't suddenly pop-up out of nowhere, announce 'I'm your advanced nurse' and have every other nurse beating a path to his or her door for support and advice. The role of an advanced nurse requires development. Nurses are a cynical lot – you have to show that you can walk the walk, not just talk the talk. Your journey to advanced or specialist practice starts as soon as you qualify.

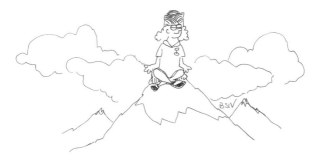

You can start preparing for specialist and advanced practice now. It doesn't matter what your career goals or aspirations are – you can work on developing the skills that will help you develop advanced practice.

Where to start?

- **First, become a reflective practitioner:** be fearless in your reflections; look at your practice, see the bad, but also see the good. Don't be less willing to accept what you do well than what you did poorly.
- **Second, develop your clinical assessment skills:** learn all you can about the areas that interest you. Don't be afraid to ask questions. Take in-service courses and training; challenge practice.
- **Third, read research and literature around your area of practice:** find someone who has a real interest and develop a professional relationship.
- **Fourth, learn to develop and listen to your insight and intuition:** learn to trust that 'gut instinct'. Develop confidence in your knowledge and your skill.
- **Fifth, and most important, commit yourself to always putting the patient first:** develop a philosophy for the care you want to give and, when you start to get stressed, go back and refocus on the philosophy: remember that patients come first.

I can hear someone out there saying 'But I just want to be a staff nurse'. The rest of you should duck, because I am about to throw something at that person.

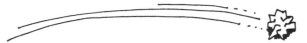

OK, the rest of us can continue now. But seriously – there is no such thing as 'just a staff nurse'. There is no one in the entire NHS more important than the nurse who, in whatever setting, delivers direct care to a patient. Even as a staff nurse you can be a leader, a teacher, an expert and someone who others come to for advice and support.

Advanced and specialist practice isn't just for academic nurses – it is something we can all aspire to. Why? Because the better prepared we are as nurses, the better care we can give and the better quality of life we can promote for our patients.

If you are interested in advanced or specialist practice, speak to someone in that role in your place of work about what he or she does. And keep reading, because throughout this book I will be giving you advice on how to be more than 'just a staff nurse'. I want you to be able to be the best nurse you can be, the nurse you want to be and the nurse your patients need you to be.

BOARDS AND COMMITTEES

You will undoubtedly be asked to be on committees, because working groups and committees are the life-blood of the health service. As a member of a committee, you have the following obligations:

- To communicate in the meeting, respectfully, waiting your turn and speaking only when you have something to say.
- To prepare by reading all the papers and getting opinions from others when it is relevant to do so.
- To undertake any actions given you in the meetings and to report on them regularly.
- To listen to others.

Boards are large committees that help to run the organisation for which you work. They are large and made up of people who are accustomed to working in high-pressure environments. But don't let that scare you – boards can also be exciting, interesting places! If you are on a board as a nurse, it is usually your place to be a voice 'for nursing'. That means that you are there to give the nursing perspective.

You behave just as you would in a committee but it's more important for you to prepare. You should research topics that are on the agenda, prepare to deliver any evidence or information about nursing related to the topics being discussed. You might need to present audit data or information from other nurses, or you might bring information back from the board and disseminate it to others in practice.

Being on a board is an honour and a huge responsibility. If you have not been involved in anything like it before, your employer should help by giving you a mentor on the board. If that doesn't happen , ask for one!

POST-QUALIFICATION EDUCATION

Most NHS organisations have programmes to help you improve your knowledge and skill. Some of these are informal, some are courses and some are programmes leading to a degree or other qualification. A common example for which someone is seconded is the district nursing course. You work for a time as a community nurse and then you are able to apply for a job in which you go to university and gain your degree and qualification.

Cost-cutting is making other kinds of support for your education less available, but not impossible. You can look into organisations that supply grants and loans if you want to fund yourself, or you can look for employment that offers you education.

If you know what you want to do, you will have a better idea of how to prepare yourself. This is yet another example of how preparing a map for your career will help: if you know you want a degree in wound care, for example, then you will start to make yourself look like the best possible candidate, so when the opportunity comes you can say 'Pick me – I'm ready!'.

You might need to fund yourself. Before you decide to do this, consider the increased earning potential. If there is none, will the course benefit you? If you choose to go down this route, consider life-learning credit: you can get credit towards a degree based on your experience, even on things you have written. For instance, do you think I wrote such a comprehensive chapter on mentorship just for this book? Perhaps I can submit it as proof that I have the knowledge and skill to get credit for a mentors and assessors course!

Be creative when looking at your life, know what you want and get credit where you deserve it. This can make it easier for you to get further education after qualification.

Look for information about loans, grants and funding awards through your professional organisation, union or university.

Summary
- Your transition from student to staff nurse might look scary but if you are a competent final-year student you will be a competent newly qualified nurse. What you think is wanted from you is far worse than what is actually wanted.
- Power and hierarchies in nursing can be frustrating, so keep focused on what is most important – your patients – and don't worry about how powerful or educated someone else might be. Concentrate on working collaboratively and your patients

will benefit. Don't gossip or play games that feed into archaic hierarchies.

- You have a wide choice of environments in which you can work: wherever you work, you must strive to be the kind of nurse who delivers the best possible care. Work in areas that you enjoy and don't let anyone tell you that you can't.
- Direct entry into community nursing is not only possible, it is increasingly becoming the norm. If you want to work in the community (or any specialist area) start to prepare as soon as you know what you want. Develop the skills and knowledge, and a pathway that will get you to the place you need to be. Don't wait until you are qualified to take the courses, in-services and self-directed training that show you are some-thing special.
- Specialist and advanced nursing is based on using your expert knowledge not just for your own practice but for others. You must have excellent communication skills, a willingness to put more effort into preparation than others and the confidence to make decisions that might not be clear cut. Being a nurse at these levels requires more education and experience but can also have more rewards.
- Know what you want from your career so you can be prepared for opportunities for further education. Be prepared to use what you have already done in your life to gain credit towards a degree or qualification. Although funding is tight, grants and loans are still available from professional bodies and unions.

POEM: *SEE ME*

This poem was found among the possessions of an elderly lady who died in the geriatric ward of a hospital. But it doesn't matter who wrote it, what matters is that the words ring true. We won't ever find out who wrote it . . . just try to make sure that no-one ever needs to write it again.

See me

> What do you see, nurses, what do you see?
> Are you thinking, when you look at me –
> A crabby old woman, not very wise,
> Uncertain of habit, with far-away eyes,
> Who dribbles her food and makes no reply,
> When you say in a loud voice – 'I do wish you'd try.'

Who seems not to notice the things that you do,
And forever is losing a stocking or shoe,
Who unresisting or not, lets you do as you will,
With bathing and feeding, the long day to fill.

Is that what you're thinking, is that what you see?
Then open your eyes, nurse, you're looking at ME . . .
I'll tell you who I am, as I sit here so still;
As I rise at your bidding, as I eat at your will.

I'm a small child of ten with a father and mother,
Brothers and sisters, who love one another;
A young girl of sixteen with wings on her feet,
Dreaming that soon now a lover she'll meet;
A bride soon at twenty – my heart gives a leap,
Remembering the vows that I promised to keep;
At twenty-five now I have young of my own,
Who need me to build a secure, happy home;
A woman of thirty, my young now grow fast,
Bound to each other with ties that should last;
At forty, my young sons have grown and are gone,
But my man's beside me to see I don't mourn;
At fifty once more babies play round my knee,
Again we know children, my loved one and me.

Dark days are upon me, my husband is dead,
I look at the future, I shudder with dread,
For my young are all rearing young of their own,
And I think of the years and the love that I've known;
I'm an old woman now and nature is cruel –
'Tis her jest to make old age look like a fool.

The body is crumbled, grace and vigour depart,
There is now a stone where once I had a heart,
But inside this old carcass a young girl still dwells,
And now and again my battered heart swells.

I remember the joys, I remember the pain,
And I'm loving and living life over again,
I think of the years, all too few – gone too fast,
And accept the stark fact that nothing can last –
So open your eyes, nurses, open and see,
Not a crabby old woman, look closer, nurses – see ME!

2 CVs and interviews

FORMATTING A PROFESSIONAL CV

What is a CV? It's your *curriculum vitae* – a Latin expression meaning 'a summary of your life' (the word 'vitae' is pronounced '**vee**-tie') and is abbreviated to CV; Americans tend to call it a *resumé*.

Your CV should not be a shopping list of everything you have ever done; it should be focused to show how well prepared you are for a particular type of work. You use your CV to show how you are the right kind of person for the kind of job you want to get. This means that although you will have a basic CV, you might want to make some minor changes, depending on the kind of job for which you are applying.

There are two aspects to consider when preparing your CV: appearance and information.

Appearance
- Good-quality paper (use something other than stark white if you can).
- Readable Sans serif typeface (Arial is a good one) in no less than size 11; 11 is the smallest easily readable font size.
- No spelling or typographical errors.
- Neat and orderly presentation.

Remember that you are a professional and there is a certain standard expected from your work. You want your CV to show that you are neat, polished and professional. Spelling and typographical errors make you look careless; a disorganised or illegible presentation will mean you never even get shortlisted.

Imagine the subtle message when your prospective employer handles a nice piece of paper after going through a stack of CVs on photocopy paper: quality. Using a lightly coloured paper also helps your CV to stand out. Together, these little details say that you took pride and spent time preparing a quality CV. Doesn't that say something important about how you would behave at work?

Information

There are two cardinal rules about what information you put onto your CV:

1. Never, ever, *ever* lie, exaggerate or 'manufacture' information in your CV.
2. Present your information in a clear, organised and sensible way.

You will need to use headings to present your information properly. Most people put them in the following order:

Name and contact details
You could head this section 'Personal details' or put the information at the top of the paper like a letterhead. Whereas your date of birth was once expected, it is no longer required in an attempt to stop age-based discrimination.

Employment
Starting with your most recent employer, work backwards and outline the last 10 years of work:

- List each job with start and finish dates (month/year). Give the employer, the general location, and your job title. List any special training, experiences or responsibilities (think about things that will illustrate your preparation for the job for which you are applying).
- You mustn't leave large gaps in your history, although it is acceptable to leave out very short-term or 'second' jobs if they don't add anything. If you had a large gap because you were doing volunteer work, put the volunteer work as a job.

EXAMPLE

Dugdown & Foundsum   Healthcare Assistant
NHS Trust   March 2004–September 2007

Achieved NVQ3 in health care. Worked with diverse client groups in general hospital. Supported nursing, medical and allied professional staff. Proficient in phlebotomy and ECG. Member of infection control committee.

Education

Start with your last formal course of study and work backwards:

- List each institution at which you studied and the dates (month/year or just year).
- List the course of study and the award given. If the award is pending you can put (pending) at the end of the entry.
- If you have taken a lot of short/certificated courses, you can list them separately at the end of the education section.
- You might want to include a separate section for awards such as A levels or NVQs.

> *EXAMPLE*
> **2004–2007 University of Middle Earth**   Dip(HE) Adult Nursing (pending)

Qualifications

Because this is a professional CV, you need to include a section about your professional qualifications:

- Give the award in your 'Education' section; in this section say what kind of nurse registration you have, when you registered, your PIN and your expiration date.
- If you are awaiting your PIN, say that it is 'pending' and give the date you applied.
- If you have taken specialist nursing courses that give you a registerable qualification, they should be listed here as well.

> *EXAMPLE*
> 2007 NMC – Adult Nurse. PIN 05Z99999Z (pending) applied September 2007.
>
> Or, for a registerable qualification other than your initial registration:
>
> 2007 NMC – Extended and Supplementary Nurse Prescriber, registered October 2007.

Achievements

If you have done anything 'special' you should have this heading.

- Published works (books/articles).
- Elected office in your nursing course, professional organisation, trade union, etc.
- Any special awards, commendations or recognition.

2005   Author, journal article 'How reflection causes brain
            damage,' published in *Journal for Cynical Students*,
            Volume 1, pp. 230–239.
2006   Author, 'Hand-washing and the student nurse: a life of
            grime,' textbook published by Baillière-Tindall.
2007   Elected Branch Chairperson, Royal College of Nursing.

Other information
List those factors that don't fit in elsewhere but could make a difference under this heading:

- languages you speak
- if you have a driving licence
- computer literacy
- your activity in a professional organisation or union (such as being a steward)
- social organisations in which you are active.

Hobbies and interests
You can use a separate heading for interests (if you want to list any). The purpose in listing interests is to show yourself as a balanced, well-rounded person. If your hobbies and interests don't do that for you, don't list them!

EXAMPLE
Other information: Full driving licence. Computer literate with Microsoft Office products and internet. Speak Urdu fluently. Union steward (Unison).
Hobbies and interests: these include history, reading, volunteering with St John's Ambulance service.

References
Who can your prospective employer contact to find out how wonderful you are? The kinds of things referees are asked about are your timekeeping, your absences, what kind of employee you were, if there were any concerns or problems about you or your work and whether the employer would hire you again. They will also be asked the dates of your employment:

- One reference will always be from your current employer: if you are at university and just qualifying, your university will be accepted as a reference. Ask who to put down as the contact person.

- The second reference should be by someone you have known more than a year, is not related to you and who knows something about your work habits and history: a previous manager, supervisor or co-worker.

Make sure you get permission *in advance* to use people as referees. Tell them you are applying for a job, remind them the kind of job you are applying for and – if necessary – remind them of the things you want to make sure they highlight in the reference.

Give the name, address, contact details and a very brief comment of why they are a referee. It is OK to list your references on a separate piece of paper; it looks neater.

Finally . . .
Keep one master copy of your CV to make sure what you put is consistent with future CVs!

If you are struggling to put your CV together, you could use the 'Wizard' in Microsoft Office, or look on the internet for some ideas. There are also many good books about preparing your CV and, often, your university will be able to give you some advice. You can even pay someone to put your CV together, but this is not usually necessary unless it's a very complicated CV and you have no idea where to start.

HOW TO APPLY FOR A JOB

First, think about what kind of job you want. Don't assume that you have to take whatever you can get – there are lots of choices out there! In Chapter 1 we discussed how to decide where you want to work; this section is about how to go through the steps of application.

So, you have decided what kind of place you want to work in. Now all you need to do is get a job and you can move on with being a nurse. There are many different places to look for job vacancies:

The internet
- Employers probably have a website that lists vacancies; call them and ask.
- There are dedicated employment websites: http://www.jobs.nhs.uk/ is the official NHS jobs website.
- The *Nursing Standard* and *Nursing Times* and Nursing and Midwifery Council websites have job listings.

Publications
- Call your local newspaper and ask which night has the best employment listings. Employers tend to advertise on a particular night each week.

- Professional journals and publications: the *Nursing Standard*, the *Nursing Times*, the *Bulletin* from the RCN, Jobs4Nurses.
- There are free employment newspapers.

Events
- Career and jobs fairs are held all over the UK, usually sponsored by a publication (such as the *Nursing Standard* or *Nursing Times*) or organisation (such as the RCN).
- There are nursing exhibitions in which potential employers have stands to promote their organisation to prospective employees.
- The NUS or your student union or university might sponsor a jobs fair.
- NHS Trusts sometimes join together for a job fair.

Go directly to the place you want to work
- You could call the human resources department of a place you would really like to work.
- You might send in a CV and covering letter asking about job openings.
- You could look out for vacancy bulletins on the wards or in the workplaces that interest you, if you are on placement there or if you know someone who works there.

Once you find out about a job, you need to make sure your CV is ready (see above).

YOUR APPLICATION

Next you need to prepare your application. Try to get two copies of the application form. If you can't, photocopy the form and use the copy as a test to make sure you complete everything properly. Hints for completing an application form:

- Use black ink.
- Print in uppercase (capital) letters.
- Be neat and legible (if you just can't, get someone to do it for you!).
- Don't abbreviate anything unless it is such a common abbreviation that it won't matter (St, Rd, etc.).
- Spell things correctly.
- Make sure the information in your application matches your CV.
- Complete the entire application: if something isn't applicable, put a line through it or write 'N/A' (for 'not applicable').

- Follow the rules: if the instruction says 'Tick this box' then tick it, even if it doesn't make sense why. Just do what the application says. If there is a guidance sheet with the application, read it *before* you put pen to the application.

Basically, your application is a reflection of you. If you can't be bothered to spell something properly, won't follow simple rules or can't be neat, then how badly do you really want that job? And how likely are employers to want you to work for them?

I have reviewed applications, and interviewed people, and I can tell you that most interviewers make the first step towards offering you a job when they read your application. I remember one of my colleagues on an interview panel saying: 'Her application was a mess – I bet her presentation is a mess, too'. That interviewer had already made her mind up. The market is tough and you don't need anyone to have a preconceived notion about you, unless it's that you are the best candidate.

YOUR PERSONAL STATEMENT

The part of the application that often throws people is the 'personal statement'. In this section, your employer is looking to answer the following question:

> *If I get 100 applications that all look the same, why should I shortlist this person rather than someone else?*

You should make sure that your personal statement covers three key areas. Now, before you read this part, I know you are probably British and ever-so unaccustomed to saying good things about yourself: this is the time to pretend that you say nice things about yourself all the time. The three key areas are:

1. Your experience, knowledge and skill relevant to this post (throw in the policies, etc. that you know are important for this post).
2. Your education relevant to this post.
3. What you expect to get out of this post, to further your career, knowledge and skill.

Think of your ideal job. Now plan your personal statement for that job. Let's look at an example. Maki has always wanted to work in elderly care. She is applying for a post as a staff nurse on a stroke rehabilitation ward.

> *I worked in a rest home from the time I was 16 until I started my nurse education, and since I started my nursing course, I have continued to work in both nursing homes and rest homes. I have*

done an NVQ3 in health care and I believe that I work very well with older people because I am patient and because I enjoy helping people regain their independence.

Because of my experience in both the nursing home and the rest home, I find that I am aware of helping patients to do things themselves, not just doing it for them. I also have excellent manual handling skills.

I would like to really develop strong rehabilitation nursing skills, especially in meeting the National Service Frameworks for Older People goals for stroke rehabilitation. I believe that the stroke service is an emerging area that has a real potential to make a difference in the lives of vulnerable people, and I would like to have an opportunity to work in that area. Eventually, I would like to work as a nurse consultant in stroke rehabilitation, so this post would be an excellent starting place for me.

The basic idea is to tell the employer why to pick you. Show that you know what's important about this post, and that you are a good match.

There is something that many people don't realise about a job advert . . . well, instead of me explaining it, read this:

Wanted: Really wanted, we need a nurse who knows what he or she is doing, who can take good care of our patients and can work well with our staff. We will give you a decent salary and support your education, and could you apply soon please? We are really struggling and need someone really good, soon!

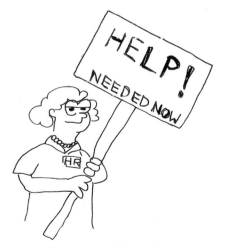

Isn't that what the average job advert really says? It's not the organisation being generous, offering you a chance and expecting you to grovel for it, it's about the organisation having a need and hoping the right person will come along to make everyone's lives easier. The organisation wants you to do it a favour – apply and fill the job. It costs thousands of pounds to have and fill a nursing vacancy – people covering the vacant post, budgets for advertising, sending out applications and letters, interviews, etc. Your potential employer wants it to be as easy as possible to fill the job with the right person.

That's why your personal statement needs to be clear about you being the right person for the job (if you are, of course!). It's so your potential employer can say 'That one will fit. Send him/her a shortlist letter'.

Another thing to think about – if you are disabled, don't hide it. Many organisations have special programmes to help disabled nurses. Look at the letterhead, organisations that display a 'double tick' have made five commitments basically assuring that not only will they interview people with disabilities, as long as they meet the minimum job requirements, but that they will continue to support disabled people in their employment through development and training. They promise to help people who develop disabilities keep their job and promise to promote awareness about disability rights in the workplace. Organisations work hard to get logos like these.

BEING SHORTLISTED

Being shortlisted is so exciting . . . you have beaten the first round and made it into the semi-finals! There is something you have to remember now: everyone that has been shortlisted is on the same ground as everyone else. It's as if you all have had the slate wiped clean and started all over again. Someone with a stunning application is going to go into the interview with theoretically the same chance as someone with their CV written in crayon (if they got shortlisted!). Remember, some interviewers start to make their mind up when they see your application but as yours looks perfect, you don't need to worry about that!

As soon as you find out you have been shortlisted, get to work.

Your preparation needs to include a general overview of the organisation you want to work for. Know what its strengths and weaknesses are: most organisations have a website that tells you demographics and targets they are working towards. Check the organisation's Healthcare Commission ratings – these will tell you some of its weaknesses! You can also ask employees about their experiences.

From this information, you need to come up with at least two questions to ask the panel. You might ask things like 'What kind of development and support is available for a new nurse in your organisation'. Write them in a notebook so you won't forget them; it's OK to write things in a notebook and read them to the panel.

- **Research the place you want to work:** find out what the mission statement and philosophy are. Is there anything really good about them? Anything really bad? Ask people who work there what kinds of things are important to the employer. Look on the website. Visit the site, if you can.
- **Find a piece of research or a journal article** that discusses something in the work area that interests you. One nurse I know brought in an article on clinical supervision in the multidisciplinary team. When the interviewer asked her 'How would you apply clinical supervision?' she took out the research article and said 'In this article, it explains . . .' and went on to briefly discuss the article and how she would apply it to her work. She knew, based on the type of job, that a question about clinical supervision would come up, so she prepared. She was not very experienced with clinical supervision and wanted to show how she was working to meet her own learning needs. It worked!
- **Plan the kinds of question you want to ask:** for example, if you were applying to work in a Trust that had been slated in the press for MRSA, you might want to ask 'What education would be available to me to help me have good infection-control practices?'. Use your questions both to determine if you really want to work there and to show your employer that you would fit in.
- **Talk to other nurses in similar jobs:** ask them what kinds of interview questions they were asked, what they do and what they think is important. This will help you think about the kinds of things the panel might ask you.
- **Know about the specialty area you are applying for:** if you are applying to work in a specialist area, such as dialysis, care of older people, the community, etc., either have relevant experience or be prepared to show that you have knowledge and interests in the area. When asked why she should get a job in dialysis, one new nurse replied 'My mother has been on peritoneal dialysis, so I know first-hand what a difference a good dialysis nurse can make for a patient and their family'. Another candidate said 'I have always had an interest in this area of nursing. I have an article here that I have been reading on the changes that have been made in dialysis machines . . . can I show you?'. If you want a job in a specialty area you are going to have to prove you have an interest in that area.

Part of your preparation also includes something about you. Have a nicely done CV ready and be prepared to give each member of the interview panel a copy. Use an attaché case or briefcase, and bring your portfolio of evidence. If you have done pertinent assignments or have testimonials, bring them. If you have written articles, had pieces published in a journal or have received any awards, bring them with you. They can't ask to see your personal portfolio but you can offer to show parts of it to them.

As well as your CV and portfolio, have mints, a notebook, two pens and a bottle of plain water.

THE INTERVIEW

First, let me tell you how interviews work . . .

An interview pro-forma will have been prepared for every candidate. On it are 10-ish questions – sometimes more, sometimes less – and each has little prompts next to it to remind the interviewers what they are looking for in the answer to that question. Candidates are asked the question by one panellist and the others make notes and write down what the candidates say, scoring against the expected and desired answers. The more closely you meet the answers that are expected by the panel, the more points you get.

Things like a presentation will count in two ways: one, you can show your knowledge about the general area; two, you demonstrate your ability to present information. You will score points in the same way as with the questions – the interviewers know what they are looking for you to say (there is more about presentations later).

After the interview, the panellists compare the scores they gave to the candidates. If it is close, they will talk about the way they feel about the different candidates and look for ways to differentiate the best candidate from the others. They will talk about their gut feelings, the candidates' demeanour, preparation and general attitude and bearing.

Getting ready for an interview

Now you know how the interview works, let's go on to how to get ready.

The final pre-interview step is to get your clothes ready. You need to try to look as though you are going to meet your partner's grandmother for the first time – conservative, neat, clean and pressed – and make sure you don't smell of cigarette smoke or heavy perfume.

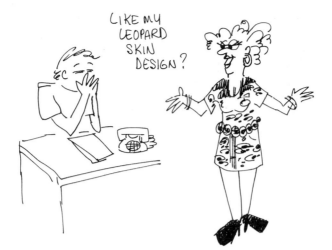

Women should wear a dress or skirt if possible, and minimise make-up. Men should wear a jacket and tie if possible. Remove or cover facial piercings: you want to appear neutral and not give the panel members anything to which they could react in a negative way.

You might be thinking 'Wait a minute . . . if they hire me, they are going to get me, so why should I hide the truth about who I am?'. The answer is that you don't want your first impression to give the wrong information about you. Someone might have an unfair bias or prejudice, or might simply feel you haven't tried very hard to look your best. Once they know you, you can relax. A good first impression in an interview is essential. You need to match their vision of the nurse they want. Worry about being an individual once you have a pay cheque.

Make sure you know how to get to the interview and do a dry run if needed. Do *not* be late. Don't eat garlic for at least 12 hours before the interview, don't eat anything you know will make you gassy, do not drink alcohol (yes, yes, I know you're nervous but . . . !) and make sure you don't smell of cigarette, cigar or any other kind of smoke. Go to the lavatory before the interview starts. Smile to yourself just before you enter the room. It will help!

During an interview

During the interview, you will probably find yourself facing a panel. One person will ask questions while the others will write. Usually, the more they write the better! Make good eye contact and try to mirror some of the interviewers' body language. This can make them see you more favourably, as long as you don't go over the top. If you don't know the answer to a question, it's OK to ask them to rephrase or ask for clarification. Make notes in your notebook about things you want to make sure to say. Don't 'uhm . . .' or 'ahh . . .'; if you need a moment to gather your thoughts, have a drink of water or just say 'Let me have a moment please . . .'. *Be warned*: if you use this pause to open a bottle of fizzy pop, it will fizz noisily, spray all over the place and embarrass you to death; that's why you bring plain water.

As you are speaking, try not to talk too fast. Don't waffle. Answer their questions as best you can. Smile. Take time to breathe.

Remember that you are doing them a favour by possibly being the person they need to do the job. It's OK to say positive things about yourself, as long as they are true! Don't ever lie: it will backfire. If you really don't know something, just admit you don't know and write the question down. Don't boast or fake it.

When the interview is finished, thank the panel. Shake hands if it feels right to do so. If you really are interested in the job, say so.

If you don't get the job, ask for feedback about your interview: they will tell you how well you did. If you are still interested, tell them: sometimes the chosen candidate won't accept the post or there might be other openings.

So, in summary: do your research and know as much as you can about the organisation and the post. Be positive about yourself, ask for clarification, dress in a conservative manner and put over a profes-sional image. Ask for feedback if you don't get the job. Interviewing is a skill, but interviews are nothing to be frightened of. Remember, you are doing the prospective employer a favour by being the nurse they need to fill their vacancy.

However . . . as well as all the above, sometimes you will be asked to give a brief presentation.

PREPARING A PRESENTATION

'I was *afraid* they were going to ask me to do a presentation!' is the plaintive cry of many a shortlisted candidate. It's the employer's chance to see if you can communicate, organise information and complete a task when requested.

You can do presentations in any manner: white board, flip chart, overhead projector or PowerPoint. Your prospective employer might specify one method. Just as when you were filling out your applica-tion, *follow the rules!*

You will usually be given a question and a limit for time. Do *not* go over the limit. The timing of a presentation is one place where less is definitely better than more.

Look at the question and think what you are really being asked. When I applied for my most recent post, the question was 'How, referring to the four key areas of the nurse consultant role, will you work to implement the National Service Frameworks for Older People'? I was given 10 minutes. It wasn't even enough time to read the title!

I looked at the question and took it apart. I discovered that the key elements were:

- the four key areas of the nurse consultant role
- the NSF for Older People
- how I would use the role to make the NSF work.

After many frenzied mind-mapping sessions, I realised that some things *weren't* part of what I was being asked:

- The interviewers didn't want me to waffle on about the NSF. If they had, I would have been given more time.
- I wasn't being asked to talk about theories but I *was* being asked to tell the interviewers what I was going to do – they said 'How *will you work* . . .' not 'What do you *think* . . .'.

So, when you get a topic for a presentation, you need to really look at what it is asking you to do. Don't think what you want to tell them – think what they have asked for.

As an example: when I was interviewing candidates for a nursing post, we asked them to tell us about nursing care for older people. One candidate did a lovely presentation about her grandmother, telling us how close she was, how ill grandma was, and so on. But she didn't say anything about nursing, and that was what we wanted to hear.

Did she get the post? What do you think?

Ten minutes is not really a very long time, if you think about it, so for my presentation I needed to plan my time carefully. I started my research. Although I was pretty sure I knew about the key roles of the nurse consultant and the NSF, I researched anyway in case I was wrong. I found good references and made notes. I thought about my experiences and my values, and what I really would do. I also like to have a good strong quote to end a presentation, so I needed to find one.

For the 10 minutes, I chose nine slides, with one of them being my introduction. You should never, ever, *ever* have as many slides as you have minutes, always less than that! At the end of this presentation, I will explain how I prepared it and prepared to give it.

Slide 1: this is the slide that I would have up when I introduced myself and gave a very brief introduction to the presentation. Just as when you do an introduction in an essay or written assignment, you need to introduce your presentation and tell

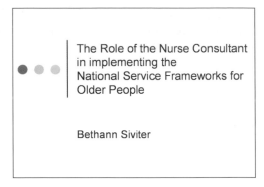

people what to expect. I told them how many slides there would be. This is important because it helps the 'audience' know when the presentation is coming to an end!

I said something like 'Thank you for allowing me to give you this presentation. In it, I will briefly look at the key areas of the nurse consultant's role, and use one specific area of the National Service Frameworks for Older People, Stroke, to illustrate the application of those key areas to the nurse consultant's work. There will be nine slides in total.'

Time so far: 45 seconds.
Time to go: 9 minutes, 15 seconds.

Slide 2: a simple outline of the four key roles.

While this slide was up, I discussed each of these roles, what they meant and how they were important in the nurse consultant role. I gave examples that showed I really did understand.

Key Roles of the Nurse Consultant

1. Expert practice
2. Professional leadership and consultancy
3. Education, training and development
4. Practice and service development, research and evaluation

Time so far: 1 minute 45 seconds.
Time to go: 8 minutes 15 seconds.

Slide 3: I then started to talk about the NSF. This slide was brief, because it was just an introduction.

I was really getting to the most important slides – and I still had enough time to explain them. It's important to limit your slides to the key points, and not to expect your slides to talk for you. It's horribly boring to have slides read to you.

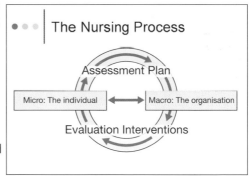

The National Service Framework for Older People

o NSF has 8 Standards
o Each standard outlines the minimum expectations for services
o Underpinned by philosophy that older people should have fair and equitable access to services that are clinically appropriate for their needs

Time so far: 2 minutes 10 seconds.
Time to go: 7 minutes 50 seconds.

Slide 4: my next slide was an outline of the NSF for Stroke. It's too complicated to outline here, but I picked out the key areas and related them to the key roles of the nurse consultant. When I was discussing this slide, I followed the order of slide 2, which outlined the key areas. First, I spoke about expert practice, then leadership, then education, then research. I mentioned that each of the Standards could be addressed by looking at them in similar ways.

Time so far: 4 minutes.
Time to go: 6 minutes.

Slide 5: the next slide was another way of looking at the way the roles would work. I explained how I saw nursing as a continuous process of assessment, planning, interventions and assessment, but that as a nurse consultant I needed to always be thinking about a wide spectrum,

The Nursing Process

Assessment Plan

Micro: The individual ⟷ Macro: The organisation

Evaluation Interventions

from the individual patient or staff person, to the entire organisation.

I did this slide because I wanted to show that I really was approaching this as a *nurse*.

Time so far: 5 minutes.
Time to go: 5 minutes.

Slide 6: my next slide was relating back to the NSFs, and how I would apply my role across the spectrum (as I described in the previous slide). I spoke about how I would work as a member of the multidisciplinary team. By now, I realised that I was being very serious, so I put in a slide next to break things up a bit.

Time so far: 6 minutes.
Time to go: 4 minutes.

Slide 7: I put this in – a variation on one of my favourite quotes. It really sums up how I feel about nursing, and I related it to my job, saying that I understood the role of the nurse consultant to be one where I would take responsibility for making sure that we offered the best care possible.

> ● ● ● | ### What really is the role of the Nurse Consultant?
>
> "Your real job as a nurse…
> If you find that something is broken,
>   then you are the one who should fix it.
> Then teach other people how to prevent
>   it from breaking again, and how to fix
>   it if it does."
>
> - Fiona Malem

This was a nice way to start my summing up. Just as in an assignment or paper, you should give a conclusion.

Time so far: 6 minutes 30 seconds.
Time to go: 3 minutes 30 seconds.

Slide 8: this next slide was just a summary. While it was up, I touched on the important points from my presentation.

> ● ● ● | ### In summary
>
> o The Nurse Consultant role has four key areas
> o These areas impact across the spectrum of care
> o The NSF is one set of guidelines with which the Nurse Consultant can guide and lead care
> o Nurse Consultancy is a process

Time so far: 7 minutes 30 seconds.
Time to go: 2 minutes 30 seconds.

Slide 9: last slide: Just another quote, to close with:

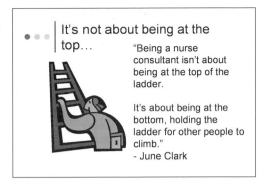

It's not about being at the top…

"Being a nurse consultant isn't about being at the top of the ladder.

It's about being at the bottom, holding the ladder for other people to climb."
- June Clark

I used this because I wanted to show that I felt the role wasn't something about power or about being important: to me, the role was (and is) about getting important work done for our patients. I spoke about my vision for the role. Then I thanked them, and asked if there were any questions.

Time so far: 8 minutes 30 seconds.
Time to go: 1 minute 30 seconds.

I handed out a copy of the slides to each member of the panel. The final slide, which I didn't show, contained all my references.

It's important to make sure that your slides are visually appealing:

- Clear, easy-to-read typeface (Arial is very good).
- Use the slide for main points, not every bit of information.
- Clear, plain slide design. It might look pretty to have black slides with white type, and a background of fireworks and stars, but it is distracting and difficult to follow the words. Use something simple.
- A logical flow of information should carry your presentation from one slide to another.
- Occasional lighter 'breaks' – using quotes, images, etc.
- Use pictures occasionally – put them on the left-hand side of the slide. The average person reads in the shape of a 'Z' – across the top from left to right, then scans across the middle, then across the bottom from left to right. Putting pictures on the left makes the slide look more balanced.
- Don't use busy or chaotic slides. Pictures should support the message that slide gives, nothing more.
- Keep animations to a minimum.
- Turn off sounds; they are too distracting.

Now let me tell you how I prepared. I made an outline of the information I wanted to convey. Remember earlier when I spoke about figuring-out what they were really asking me? That is where my outline started. I took the elements of the question:

- The four key areas of the nurse consultant role.
- The NSF for Older People.
- How I would use the role to make the NSF work.

My outline looked like this:

1. *Give introduction.*
2. *Outline the four key areas of the role.*
3. *Introduce the NSF for older people.*
4. *Pick one area to use as an illustration.*
5. *Explain the micro to macro nature of the role.*
6. *Show how the nursing process underpins the role.*
7. *Give a quote or two to show how I really feel about the role.*
8. *Summarise.*
9. *Give a good close: leave them something to think about.*

If you look back, each of these turned into a part of my presentation.

Remember: your outline is crucial for getting your presentation right. It's the road map – turn left, turn right, arrive at your destination. Without a map, you will get lost, and lost is not where you want to be.

I took 4 × 6-inch record cards (index cards). I wrote one part of the outline on each card, then did some research and decided what order I wanted them in, and what I wanted on the slides. It helped me decide how much information to put on one slide – the cards are about the right size.

Once I knew what each slide should have, I worked on my presentation. I found a nice background and put the slides together. Then I printed the slides off, six slides to a page as handouts. I took new index cards and pasted one slide on each card. Using my old cards for reference, I wrote out what I wanted to say. I like to use bullet points, but some people like to have a whole script.

I added notes like 'Pause for a breath!' 'Smile' and so on to remind me not to rush and to help me with my nerves.

Once I had my cards, I practised in front of a clock to check my timing. I wanted to leave a minute at the end to give me room in case there was a problem with a slide, or if someone asked me a question.

Remember: practice makes perfect: you need to be as comfortable and confident about your information as possible. You need to be able to recite it forwards and backwards. Don't be intimidated – it doesn't take long. Just practise. Keep the cards to remind you, but – if you prepare – when the time comes the words will just flow and you will make a great impression. If you don't prepare, it will show. How badly do you want that job?

I then wrote a rough guideline of how much time it would take on the cards. Now all I had to do was practise, practise, practise and practise some more. Any friend who didn't know better was sucked into listening to my presentation. I did it over and over until it felt comfortable.

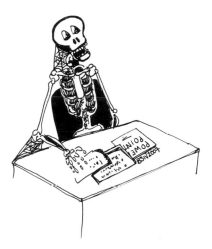

Along the way, I fixed a few things, changed a few things and took a few things out.

By the time I went to give it, I could recite it backwards if I had to! This allowed me to focus on my body language and posture and not worry about tripping over words.

Presentations can be intimidating but they can also be fun. Just think – it's 10 fewer minutes you have to worry about answering questions! A good presentation can make the difference between a job offer and a 'thanks-but-no-thanks' letter. It's the chance for you to shine, show how passionate and knowledgeable you are, and make a real impression. Just make sure you understand what they want, outline it so you have the road map, don't put in too many slides, make the slides easy to read – and practise!

STANDING OUT IN A CROWD

Today's reality is that there are often more nurses than there are posts, so you have to make sure you have that special something that the employer wants.

● Does your CV – honestly and completely – reflect your best points?

- Will your referees give the best view of you, and will they say 'Hire her, she's worth it'?
- Are you prepared to sell yourself as the best candidate?
- Are you prepared to do the type of nursing role for which you are applying?

If you can answer 'Yes' to all of these, you are starting in a good place. However, a subsequent problem will be making sure that the panel knows you are best for the job. How do they determine who is best?

- The one who gives the best most complete answers: if you think you need to keep answering a question, keep talking. Think for a moment before you answer and don't be afraid to expand on your answers.
- Show evidence of your preparation for the interview: don't be afraid to say something like 'I thought a long time before I applied for this post – I thought "Can I be the nurse they need" . . .' Show the panel you are thoughtful and considerate.
- Show evidence of skill: have you attended seminars and training? Have you taken advantage of development opportunities? Have you written for a publication? Even a letter to the editor? How are you better prepared than another nurse might be? Even personal experience matters: 'I took care of my grandmother . . .' is better than 'No' when asked if you have experience caring for the elderly, for example.

The last points. Smile. Look neat. Be tidy. Be on time. Smell good. Be personable. The panel wants to hire the nurse who can not only do the job but will be someone others want to work with; the interviewers don't just want a nurse who will work hard, they want a nurse who will work well with others.

Standing out in a crowd is something that takes preparation, time and forethought. You can't do it on a moment's notice. You need to put time into being the nurse the panel wants you to be, and be willing to blow your own trumpet so they notice.

You will get a nursing job; you might not get the one you want but eventually you will be working in the area you want to work in. Don't give up; learn from your experiences (reflect even!) and keep trying.

Summary
- A good CV is honest, well thought out and well presented.
- Use good-quality paper and a clear typeface.
- Apply for jobs you *want*.
- Fill in your application neatly in black ink.

- Prepare for your interview by learning as much as you can about the job and the organisation.
- Make the best possible first impression.
- Ask for feedback if you are unsuccessful.
- If asked to prepare and deliver a presentation, prepare and practise to get it right.
- You need to stand out as the best candidate: don't be afraid to tell the panel how you stand out.

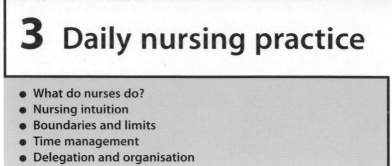

3 Daily nursing practice

- What do nurses do?
- Nursing intuition
- Boundaries and limits
- Time management
- Delegation and organisation
- Summary
- References

There is a debate in nursing: is it an art or a science? Most people claim it's both, but to varying degrees. I think of it this way: if you are an artist who paints portraits in oils, then science – knowing what paints to use, how to use them, your technical ability and skill – is what you use to express your art. Your artistic ability is what guides you to use your technical skills; the technical skills allow you to express your art. The two go hand in hand.

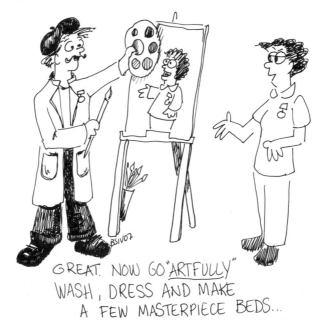

GREAT. NOW GO "ARTFULLY"
WASH, DRESS AND MAKE
A FEW MASTERPIECE BEDS...

In this chapter and the next, we will be looking at some of the art underpinning nursing practice. The science – your technical skills and abilities – is one thing: the art – having vision and an understanding of *why* we do what we do – is another, and is often neglected in preparation and support for nurses.

If you know how to make decisions, and how to think like a nurse, then you will be well on the road to being the nurse you need to be.

WHAT DO NURSES DO?

According to Henderson (1966):

Nursing is primarily assisting the individual in their performance of those activities contributing to health, or its recovery that they would perform unaided if they had the necessary strength, will, or knowledge.

Recently, the Royal College of Nursing (RCN 2003) defined nursing as:

The use of clinical judgement in the provision of care to enable people to improve, maintain, or recover health, to cope with health problems, and to achieve the best possible quality of life, whatever their disease or disability, until death.

To really understand these, we first need to look at what 'health' is. A search for 'health' on the internet leads to some diverse opinions:

- being free from disease or illness
- the ability to cope with everyday activities
- a state of balance
- ability to survive
- a social situation with rewarding relationships
- being financially solvent
- being without stress or worry
- complete physical, mental and social well-being
- free from abnormality
- free from abuse or exploitation
- being able to enjoy and participate in activities.

So, what *is* health? If it is an ability to survive then a baby isn't healthy because it relies on someone else to meet its needs. Is it the absence of disease or illness? Well, that definition would make it impossible for anyone with a chronic disease to ever aspire to health. What about the ability to cope? I can cope with some things well and other things (like approaching book deadlines . . .) a little less well. I don't know about you, but for me coping is relative.

That's the real key to 'health' – health is relative. Health is the relationship between your potential (ability to cope, to have relationships, to function physically and psychologically) and actual states. The closer your potential is to your actual status, the healthier you are.

If you were a 90-year-old woman with arthritis, high blood pressure and diabetes, would you be 'healthy'? What if you were still able to get out and do your shopping, you were able to live with your arthritis because of appropriate medication, your diabetes and blood pressure were diet controlled and you still had social activities that you enjoyed?

Would you, as that woman, be less or more healthy than a 40-year-old man who is stressed by working too many hours, smokes, drinks and is a little overweight, even though he doesn't have high blood pressure, arthritis or diabetes?

Health is relative. As a nurse, it's your job to help improve individuals' potential health and bring their actual state closer to their potential state. If the best a patient can have for a healthy life is to be cared for around the clock and enjoy social interaction by watching television, then that's health, for that person.

Your nursing assessment needs to identify your patient's actual and potential states of psychological, physical and social health. Your assessment is the foundation of holistic care: looking not just at the body, or the mind, but at the life of the individual.

By understanding health, being able to assess health potentials and acting to promote, maintain and restore the individual's health potential, you are *nursing*. It's not something you can do with a written model, a document, a pill or a blood-pressure cuff. Nursing is using what you know and – to some extent – who you are, to help patients and their carers find and remain in the place they need to be.

NURSING INTUITION

What is nursing intuition:

- A strange psychic ability?
- Lucky guessing?
- What you get from your nursing tutor?
- Awareness developed as a result of reflection, experience and education?

Intuition is that feeling you get without knowing why you get it. It happens to every nurse at every level: it's that little voice inside you:

I only just qualified as a children's nurse, but I have had four children of my own and now even a grandchild. When I was working one night, I couldn't help but think there was something wrong with this one little lad. His obs were fine, nothing seemed obvious, but this little voice kept telling me to pay attention. I checked him far more frequently than I would usually. On one check I realised he was sweating. I took his temperature – his skin was hot – and found it very high. To make a long story short, he had a serious infection but we were able to treat him quickly. I don't know how I knew; I just did.

This story is not unique: you hear it all the time:

- 'I just knew'
- 'I had this funny feeling'
- 'Something just told me'.

Sometimes, it's about simple things:

I just decided to swab the wound; it didn't look really infected, just a bit inflamed, but I just thought it was a good idea. Turned out to be infected with MRSA.

Sometimes, more complicated things:

The night nurse called the family and suggested they come in. Their mother was dying but the doctors thought it was still a matter of at least a week. The night nurse just felt that it would be a good idea for them to come in. The patient passed away an hour or so after they got here.

How do nurses know? Where does that 'funny feeling' come from? Some people say it's an instinct with some kind of psychic basis, but most people agree that intuition in nursing is the result of cues that the nurse isn't consciously aware of. Looking at the examples above, how could the nurses have known?

The nurse who swabbed the wound and found MRSA: perhaps there was a certain odour or appearance that the nurse had seen many times before that always turned out to be MRSA or some other infection. The nurse probably realised unconsciously that:

This smell + that appearance = MRSA.

As a result of this conclusion, the nurse decided to swab the wound.

The nurse who knew, without knowing why, that the family should come in had worked nights for years. How many dying patients had she cared for? She probably recognised, unconsciously, the cues and signals that meant the patient was going to die soon.

What we know for sure that these occurrences have in common is that the nurses had experience and were aware enough to hear and listen to those inner voices. That experience isn't just nursing experience. The life you had before you became a nurse (LBN = life before nursing) gave you valuable knowledge and skills: don't underestimate its importance. Part of your process of development as a nurse is learning how to relate your LBN to your life as a nurse.

Think about some of the skills and knowledge you bring:

- You have had relationships and interactions with many different people.
- You have been a partner/spouse/child.
- You have been a student.
- You have had experiences in different working environments.
- You have had personal and family health worries.
- You have had good days and bad days.
- You have been filled with grief, joy, worry, pain and fear.
- You have been lazy and motivated.

Each of us brings different experiences to nursing and these experiences, as they integrate into practice, will influence the nurse we become.

Think for a moment about a jigsaw puzzle. When you first begin, you identify the edge pieces and you group the colours together. As you start to work the puzzle, you might notice that certain subtle tones (for an example, let's use the colour blue) are more common in one place than another. Using nothing more than that, you start to further separate blue pieces from other blue pieces. Someone with less experience in puzzles might not realise that this is a useful strategy; he or she might use more trial and error.

The more experience you have, the less you need to use trial and error and the more quickly, and accurately, you can put the puzzle pieces together. It's the same in nursing.

As you reflect (see Chapter 6), you start to integrate who you are as a person – your beliefs, feelings, knowledge and past experience – into your nursing practice. As you begin to reflect 'in action' rather than just 'on action' this integration of experience and knowledge will start to become more unconscious. This is where you will start to really develop your intuition. As you read research, learn more about evidence-based practice and add to your knowledge, skill and experience base, the resources for your unconscious decision-making will grow.

With further reflection, you learn to hear that 'little voice' from your unconscious awareness. You will probably find, as most experienced nurses have, that you often regret not listening to that inner voice.

In *The student nurse handbook* (Siviter 2004) I explain a little about 'Nurse Brain', how being a nurse affects the way you think for the rest of your life. You don't see things the same any more: you notice when someone looks unwell, you think more about health and health-related issues, you can't help but relate to the world as a nurse. 'Nurse Brain' is really when you allow reflection and intuition to be tools you use every day: you can be a nurse without reflection and intuition but these elements make you a better nurse than you could ever be without them.

There is much more to being a nurse than just providing hands-on care. Nursing is a profession in which nurses themselves use their nursing knowledge and skill to make decisions: they use their highly tuned 'Nurse Brain' to guide what they do and how they do it. Nurses who develop and listen to their intuition are more sensitive to patients, families and their needs. They are more likely to solve a problem before it gets out of control, and less likely to make mistakes.

In *From novice to expert*, Benner (2001) gives a very concrete path for the development of expertise in nursing, and recognises that the development of intuition is not just an element of development but a hallmark of nursing expertise. Personally, I don't think the development is as concrete as Benner relates but I do believe that, to become expert, you need to be an intuitive and reflective practitioner.

This intuition is why experienced nurses can use their expertise as evidence for evidence-based practice. Sometimes, an experienced nurse says 'I just *know*, that's why'. If you don't develop that inner voice, then a huge area of nursing practice and expertise will be closed to you.

BOUNDARIES AND LIMITS

There are two parts to boundaries and limits: respecting them and making sure other people respect yours. In Chapter 5 we will talk about assertiveness; in this chapter we will talk about how you respect the boundaries and limits of your own practice.

Boundaries

Poor boundaries in nursing often result when we are more concerned about getting our own needs met than meeting our patient's needs. The Nursing and Midwifery Council's (NMC's) *Code of professional conduct* tells us that we must have good boundaries, that we must not abuse the power our position gives us and that we must work to protect the public, not be someone they need protection from. These are key principles to being professional and are at the very core of professional behaviour: it's these boundaries that help us behave in a professional way.

Having poor boundaries – often called 'behaving in an unprofessional manner' – will cause trouble for you, personally and professionally. Nurses are caring people who work very closely with often quite vulnerable people, and it is easy for boundaries to blur. But you have an obligation to keep boundaries clear.

What are good boundaries?
- Not overstepping the line between professional and personal relationships.
- Being able to say 'No' when it's appropriate.
- Always putting the patient and the patient's needs before your own.
- Making certain that you act in a way that maintains trust and upholds the reputation and image of nursing and nurses.

Some simple ways to keep good boundaries
- **Don't give patients your personal contact details.**
- **Don't ever keep a 'secret':** as a professional, you must work with the team. Don't flatter yourself into thinking that you have a 'special' relationship with a patient. If the patient speaks to you it can't be a secret because it's part of your professional role to communicate with others in the team. Secrets are something you tell friends, not healthcare professionals.
- **Do *your* job:** you have to know what things are your responsibility to take care of and what things aren't. If your patient is in a domestic abuse situation but you are not her counsellor or social worker, then you shouldn't try to do the counsellor's or social worker's job. Focus on doing your job and supporting others in theirs, not trying to do their job for them.
- **Don't tell too much about yourself:** it is not appropriate to focus your interactions on yourself. Let me give you an example: I have an obvious American accent and patients often ask where I am from. I can't really say 'Let's not talk about me . . .' it would seem rude. So, I tell them where I am from and ask them where *they* are from. I try to move the conversation around to get them talking about themselves. Would I love to stand there and chat non-stop about America? Probably. But that's not what I am there for.

Because nursing becomes such an important part of you it's hard to forget that you are a nurse. It's important, though, because to be healthy (having a balance between social and working lives) means having time for you. If you never have time for yourself, you will start to steal time for yourself from your work time: bad boundaries result.

Those bad boundaries can take away opportunities to relax and enjoy life. I let it slip on one glorious holiday that I was a nurse and I spent a week listening to people talk on and on about their constipation, bunions and tablets. It wasn't fun. Worse, though, because they knew I was a nurse I knew I had to be careful how I answered their questions. They would see me as an expert, whether I was really an expert or not. I tried to be assertive and not be their personal nurse/health advisor but once you open the door some people can be very persistent!

Boundaries are also very important to your co-workers
The things you do will set a precedent for other staff. Your behaviour can teach your patients what to expect from nurses and other staff. If you always bring them a chocolate bar from home they might start to wonder why others don't.

If you find yourself doing 'extras' for patients, you need to look closely at your behaviour:

- Are there certain kinds of patients for whom you do extras and some for whom you don't?
- Are you setting up unfair expectations that other staff might have to cope with?
- Are you treating the patient with dignity and respect?
- What are your motives? Be really honest with yourself: is this about the patient or about trying to look good?

You have an obligation under the NMC *Code of professional conduct* to treat everyone fairly, with respect. This means that you must treat all your patients the same. Can you do extras for everyone? If other patients knew what you were doing, might they feel that they are being treated unfairly?

In all honesty, there are times we all 'break the rules'. For example, as a district nurse, very occasionally I would give a patient a lift to an appointment. I made sure she knew I was not doing this as her nurse and I told her it was not something to expect again! But I had a dilemma – the patient *badly* needed to see the consultant, transport was very late and she didn't have the taxi fare. What could I do? I could have paid for the taxi, perhaps, but I had to get her to the appointment somehow.

The point is that I thought about it, about the risks for me and for my patient, and I decided that the patient needed me to do this because it was the right thing *for her*. To be honest, it made me very nervous. I can be absolutely certain that I did it for her, not me! And, when it was over, I spoke to my manager about it. To her credit, she quizzed me on my motives and we came to the conclusion that in this isolated incident I did the right thing.

That's the other thing about boundaries – never do anything that you might feel you can't tell your manager. If you can't tell others what you have done, you probably shouldn't be doing it.

Certain vulnerable groups can be seriously affected by a nurse's failure to keep good boundaries. People with learning disabilities, those with mental illness, children and older people are more likely to be hurt or confused by one nurse behaving one way and others behaving differently. In some cases, this confusion might lead to aggression or inappropriate behaviour from the patient – let me give you an example.

A nurse I will call Deb was working in a home for people with learning disabilities. She felt really badly for one of the lads there, David: his family refused to buy him cigarettes and he was always borrowing them from other residents. Because of his behavioural issues, he wasn't able to go to a shop and buy them himself. So Deb started to loan David a cigarette here and there. And then she started buying him an occasional pack. One day she overheard two clients squabbling: when she got to the bottom of it she realised that her relationship with David had got out of control. David had told other clients that Deb was his girlfriend and was arguing with other clients whenever he felt that one of them was trying to get her attention. Simple friendship had been misinterpreted and had caused distress for David and for others. The next few weeks, as things were sorted out, were very stressful and unpleasant for everyone.

It would have been better if Deb had spoken to her manager about the cigarettes and found a way for David to buy them for himself.

Limits

Limits are very closely related to boundaries but are more related to competence and knowledge than to interpersonal issues.

The NMC *Code of professional conduct* tells you very clearly that you must recognise the responsibility you have to the public as a whole and to each individual patient. You are fully accountable for the way you behave and the actions you take. You are accountable for being prepared to do your job, academically, technically and emotionally. If you are not ready to practise, you have an obligation to tell someone and get help. These things are key to setting and keeping limits.

Respecting limits means knowing your professional boundaries. As a nurse, you have an obligation to:

- Know what you are competent to do, and work to maintain your competency.
- Know what you aren't competent to do, and work to become competent.
- Not try to do what you know you aren't competent to do.
- Seek support from someone who *is* competent as you learn.

The bottom line, as with everything, is that patients, their families and carers must have faith in you. That doesn't mean they expect you to know and be able to do everything – they expect you to do what you can do well, and get help for everything else.

If you are trying very hard to be the best nurse you can be, as I imagine you are (or you would not have bought this book!) it's not always easy to say 'I can't do that' and ask for help. As a reflective practitioner (see Chapter 6), you should already be aware of your skills and limitations, but feeling like you have to ask for help – especially when other people are busy – is something most nurses like to avoid. Your colleagues might be a bit stressed the moment you ask them for help but, in the long run, we all need help from each other. Don't ever be too shy, ashamed or proud to ask for help.

TIME MANAGEMENT

Forget blood pressures, assessments and every other technical nursing skill you have learned: time management is one of the two most important skills you will ever use in nursing. The other – communication – is discussed in Chapter 5. (Don't *really* forget that other stuff, by the way, I was only making a point.)

If you can't organise and manage your time, you won't get everything done. Nursing is stressful and filled with interruptions and ever-changing priorities. How can you make sure it all gets done? By knowing what you need to do, when you need to do it.

Time management happens at two levels: what I call 'micro' (the small level) and 'macro' (the bigger level). Let me give you an example:

> If I have to do three patient assessments and an audit, I have different planning and time frames for each. On the 'micro' level: I have to do the assessments today, this shift. There isn't a lot of planning. The audit is more at the 'macro' level: it's beyond this one shift, although I might do parts of it on this shift. It requires a more in-depth planning that might include other people; the micro-level planning affects me, and this shift, only.

When you are looking ahead at your work for the day, take a moment to consider how you can meet as many needs as possible. For example, you are helping me with my audit (thank you so much!), you have three patients who need dressing changes and one who needs a continence assessment (in addition to everything else that all our patients need). You know that my audit is around continence so, as you do the assessment, you also complete the audit form. Combining the micro and macro helps to get everything done.

Time management also means cleaning up after yourself. OK, prepare for a rant: no-one has the right to put needless work onto anyone else. You made it dirty? You clean it. You took the wrong thing from the equipment room? You put it back. Don't leave anything else . . . actually, let me pause here and wash up the coffee mug I left on the sink in the kitchen. Be right back (musical intermission). OK, what was I saying? Oh yes. Keep things tidy, put things back where they belong and you won't have to interrupt other things because you need to clean-up or look for something that has been misplaced.

Good time management

There are some cardinal rules for good time management:

- Know what you need to get done.
- Know when potential problems, such as interruptions or even just your own habits, will make things difficult.
- Know when you can be flexible and when you can't.
- Have strategies for coping with problems as they occur.
- Don't make extra work for yourself (or anyone else) through untidiness, lack of organisation or laziness.
- Being stressed reduces your ability to think, and a reduced ability to think doesn't help you get things done.
- Plan ahead.

How can you plan ahead?

Try an experiment: for the next seven shifts, log everything you do and how much time you spend. Every time you change activity, enter it in. Be honest. It would be useful to prepare the log and headings in advance. You could use the following:

- Activity
- Start
- Finish
- Time allocated
- Time actually spent

- How you were feeling
- Time-wasters.

This leads you to the next step of keeping a time log: analysing your time patterns. Once you have a number of days logged, look at the records:

- Identify the things you do every day: how much time on average is spent on each one?
- How do your feelings change with different tasks? Are there certain times of the day that you are tired, stressed, etc.?
- How often do you spend only the allocated time on an activity? How often do you go over?
- What are main time-wasters – interruptions, chatting, looking for something?

Table 3.1

Activity	Start	Finish	Time allocated	Time actually spent	How were you feeling?	What were the 'time-wasters'?
Handover	8.00	8.40	30 min	40 min	Tired	Chatted for a few minutes with the night staff
Quick ward check	9.00	9.30	30 min	30 min	Irritated at things that hadn't been done	No, well, yes, complaining to others
Drug rounds	9.30	11.00	1 hour	90 min	Stressed	Kept being interrupted
Break	11.00	11.20	10 min	20 min	Glad to be off the ward	Kept talking to another staff member

Then think of things you can do to solve some of the problems you have found:

- Is there anything you can delegate or simplify?

- Can you reorganise your work pattern or schedule?
- Can you get help from other people?
- Where do the time-wasters come from, and are there any I can eliminate?

Let's look back at the examples:

Table 3.2

Activity	Start	Finish	Time allocated	Time actually spent	How were you feeling?	What were the 'time-wasters'?
Handover	8.00	8.40	30 min	40 min	Tired	Chatted for a few minutes with the night staff
Quick ward check	9.00	9.30	30 min	30 min	Irritated at things that hadn't been done	No, well, yes, complaining to others

On a quick ward check, you might make sure that everyone has their nurse call light, water, etc., and make sure that supplies and equipment is ready for the day ahead. Between handover and the ward check, this nurse has spent 70 minutes and is frustrated by things that weren't done, adding to her stress for the day. Also, look at the gap between 8.40 and 9.00. What do you think was happening then? The nurse was probably delegating to other staff.

What if this nurse proposed a change to handover, by having one member of staff do a quick ward check with a member of staff from the night before, while the other members of staff did handover. At the end of the check, the two could compare notes, join the handover meeting and then delegate whatever needed to be delegated. The nurse in handover gathers the information and the staff member on the ward check might highlight areas that were left undone the night before. Maybe it isn't even a nurse who needs to do the ward check.

OK, look at the next part of the example:

Table 3.3

Activity	Start	Finish	Time allocated	Time actually spent	How were you feeling?	What were the 'time-wasters'?
Drug rounds	9.30	11.00	1 hour	90 min	Stressed	Kept being interrupted
Break	11.00	11.20	10 min	20 min	Glad to be off the ward	Kept talking to another staff member

This nurse started the drug rounds stressed (you know this from the time log from the ward check). Perhaps, seeing that being interrupted has wasted half an hour, she proposes that the nurse doing the drug rounds shouldn't be interrupted. It is safer for medication administration and would help the nurse get it done more quickly so that patients get their medication on time.

By looking at what you do, when and how long it takes, you can get an overall picture of when things go wrong. You can't always fix things but you can work on coping with the problems you encounter. By identifying problems – in your own practice and with others – you are moving towards solving those problems. Never just complain or know there is a problem and do nothing: if it's important enough to whine about, it's too important not to fix. (The moral of the story: she who doesn't wish to solve problems shouldn't whine!)

Logging your time can also give you a picture of the organisation of the activities during the shift. For example, do you frantically work to get everyone up, washed and sitting in a chair by 11.00 a.m. and then consistently have a slow hour or so around 1 and 2 in the afternoon? Would it be better, perhaps, to save a bath or two until the early afternoon and make the morning less frantic? You might not recognise these patterns until you take the time to look for them: that's what the time log is for.

Time management links in very closely with organisation and delegation. You can't manage your time properly without them.

DELEGATION AND ORGANISATION

Delegation is sharing out your work with other people; organisation is how you organise your day and your workload to get everything done in a timely way. If you organise your work, you can see what things you need to delegate. Does that make sense?

Let's talk about delegating things first.

Rule one: one person – with one brain and one set of hands – can't do everything

- You will need to prioritise: what can only be done by you and what others can do safely and appropriately.
- You will need to choose which tasks can wait until later and which must be done now.

Delegating is one of the more challenging tasks you will have. It can cause tension and stress, and some nurses prefer to do too much rather than ask anyone to help them (read the section called 'The smell of burning martyr' in Chapter 8). So, to decide what to delegate, ask yourself:

- What can only a qualified member of staff do? That is, legally, ethically, professionally, according to Trust policy.
- Does this task require a nursing judgement or skilled intervention?
- Does the person I might delegate this to have the necessary knowledge and skill?
- If it is delegated, how badly could things go wrong?
- Does the person to whom I delegate this have the support he or she needs?
- Am I being lazy by asking someone else to do it?
- Is there anything to make me think it should not be delegated?
- What is the best use of my time, for my patient's best interest?

The answers to these questions will help you decide what you can delegate and what you should do yourself.

Delegating starts with knowing what you have ahead of you for the day. In handover, make a note of all the things that have to be accomplished. Organising your day starts here. Imagine the following:

There are 25 beds on your ward. There are two trained nurses and two HCAs working with you, although one of the HCAs goes home at midday. You also have a second-year student. It's 8.00 a.m.

To make handover most effective, you should be prepared. Have a list of the basic information about each patient and use handover to gather new information.

Table 3.4

Bed	Patient name/age	Doctor	Problem/ diagnosis	Notes
1	Agatha Crusty, 68	Rowe	Falls? syncope (fainting) or TIA (transient ischaemic attack)	Clinic appointment tomorrow ☐ Book transport
2	Melinda Marple, 80	Dunstan	Fractured L neck of humerus	☐ Discharge today ☐ L shin dressing
3	Clarisse Clouseau, 77	Goodman	Left total hip replacement	Possible UTI ☐ MSU ☐ Nutritional assess.
4	Jane Bond, 79	Mayer	CVA L side	☐ MRI today ☐ Pressure area care
5	Jennifer Fletcher, 80	Main	L above knee amputation, diabetes	☐ Dressing OT doing home visit
6	Parminder Patel, 67	Turnbull	New type 2 diabetes, leg ulcers	☐ Dressings ☐ BM

During handover, start to identify things that need to be done and put a little box or circle that you can tick when it's done. This gives you a handy 'to-do' list.

For these six patients, in addition to all the essential care (beds, baths, obs, etc.) you have:

- transport to be booked
- a discharge
- four dressings
- a BM (blood monitoring)
- a patient going on a home visit
- an MSU (midstream urine sample)
- a nutritional assessment.

What things can only you do? What can be delegated? Are there things that can be done at the same time as other things? What are your priorities? Go through your list (the extra columns aren't part of your handover, they are the things that you should be thinking in your head).

As you do, remember the following:

- What things will probably interrupt me, and how can I plan ahead for them?
- What things can wait until later?
- What is the best use of my time?
- How can I appropriately use delegation?

Table 3.5

Bed	Activity	Think	Action
1	Clinic appointment tomorrow ☐ Book transport	Do you have to book transport or can you delegate this?	Delegate to ward clerk
2	☐ Discharge today ☐ L shin dressing	You need to get the dressing done before she goes home, and you need to send dressings home for the District Nurse. Is all the discharge paperwork done? Does the patient have everything from pharmacy?	Get all the dressings together, for this change and for home Do this dressing first Need to make sure everything is ready for the discharge
3	Possible UTI ☐ MSU ☐ Nutritional assessment	When do I need the MSU? When can I do the assessment? Can I combine any of these?	Delegate MSU to an HCA Plan to observe how much she eats at breakfast and lunch, will do assessment after lunch
4	☐ MRI today ☐ Pressure area care	What time is the MRI? What time will transport come? Does anything need to be ready? When can I do the pressure area care?	MRI: patient needs notes and old films Appointment at 1.00 p.m. Pressure areas will be affected by transport: do them now
5	☐ Dressing OT doing home visit	Does this dressing need to be done now, or can it wait until after OT? Will it be too late for me to do the dressing then? How does the patient feel?	Find out when home visit will take place Speak with patient – does she want dressing changed first

Table 3.5

Bed	Activity	Think	Action
6	☐ Dressings ☐ BM	What time do you need the BM? Can you delegate this? When does the dressing need to be done?	Speak with nursing student: is student interested in doing BM and some diabetic teaching? Do dressing afternoon

New things will pop up during your working day and demand a place on your 'to do' list. If you always know which things can wait, you know where you can put new problems on the list. One way to know what things can wait is to 'triage' things on your list.

Triage means sorting things out depending on how urgent they are. I use an 'ABCD' system:

- **A**: absolutely must get done before other things.
- **B**: better get done sooner rather than later.
- **C**: can wait until later.
- **D**: don't worry about it.

Absolutely must get done . . .

These are the things that must be done before you can really concentrate on doing other things; things that if you don't do them now someone is going to interrupt you to do them while you are doing something else. These are things other people might be waiting for before *they* can carry on: in the above example, it could be doing a dressing while patient transport is wasting time waiting for me.

Better get done sooner . . .

These are the things that, although not life or death, are important and need to get done. Although no one will die if you leave them in bed an extra half an hour, it is unpleasant to be left stuck in bed, so you must get people up, washed and dressed after you have done all the things that can't wait. Sometimes, you can do some 'Better get done's' while waiting for opportunities to get 'Absolutely' tasks finished; for example, if you need a urine sample (an 'absolutely') take the time to get the person to the loo and get washed at the same time.

Can wait until later . . .

These are the 'when you have a chance' things. Things like going to the pharmacy to get something not needed until the afternoon. Some paperwork and administrative tasks are 'can waits'. You have to make sure they get done but you can fit them in whenever there is time.

Don't worry about it . . .

Some things are nice to do but, if you don't get them done, it won't affect your patient care. Things like putting together documents in advance for new admissions or stocking for the next shift – you get the general idea.

When making your 'to-do' list, rank things according to my ABCD list. Don't worry about Bs until all the As are done. If you suddenly find a new task, rank it according to its priority.

Let's put ABCD on the tasks you already have identified:

Table 3.6

Bed	Activity	Priority?
1	Clinic appointment tomorrow ☐ book transport **A**	**A**: Pass over to clerk as soon as she gets in
2	☐ L shin dressing **A** ☐ Discharge today **A**	**A**: Otherwise, transport will be here and I will have to rush to change the dressing and get things ready **A**: Make sure everything is ready for discharge. Ask clerk to check first thing and let me know before 9.30
3	Possible UTI ☐ MSU **A** ☐ Nutritional assess. **B**	**A**: Yes, labs need to go early **B**: Make sure I ask someone to observe for me if I am not there
4	☐ MRI today **A** ☐ Pressure area care **A**	**A**: Yes: Don't want to get interrupted. Will delegate getting records and old films to clerk **A**: Will do pressure care first thing
5	☐ Dressing **A or B or C** OT doing home visit	**A**: Have to know what time and how patient feels: these have to happen right away so I can plan what to do. Then I can decide if this is A, B or C
6	☐ Dressings **A** ☐ BM **C**	**A**: Prioritise speaking to student nurse to see if she is able to do this **C**: Dressing is low priority but must be done today

So you have your basics. A bunch of As and Bs, one C (the column was just to help you visualise what you should be thinking). How would this list change if:

- The MRI was cancelled: would the pressure-area care still be an A?
- The woman needing the nutritional assessment went into cardiac arrest: is the nutritional assessment still something to worry about?
- The discharge was delayed until tomorrow: is the dressing still an A?
- Mrs Patel in bed 6 fell and needed an urgent X-ray: are there other things more or less important than getting the X-ray sorted? Would you do a BM before she went off to X-ray or when she returned?
- What if the student nurse didn't know how to do a BM? Do you have the time to teach her?

As things change, you might need to re-prioritise. Be flexible, adapt to things as they change and you will find it much easier.

It takes time and practice to get used to organising your work for a shift. Watch the way others do it. If you find some people who always seems to have things under control, ask how they organise themselves and learn from them. Some nurses use coloured ink; others use little lists. With experience, nurses develop ways to plan their time. You will too. If you don't, your job will be very stressful and you won't be able to give the best care possible.

You need to consider more than just your own time. Think about when other staff want to take breaks, and when staff go home or come in. Think about how it must feel to wait when you are unwell. If you know something needs to be done between 10 and 10.30 a.m., don't ask someone who takes their break at 10 – you will stress them and it might not get done.

That brings us back to delegating. I bet you were hoping I had forgotten but I had it on my list as a 'B'!

The best way to minimise stress is to use your best interpersonal skills when delegating:

- Tell the person, specifically, what you need done and when it needs to be done.
- Ask – don't order – politely and with respect.
- Consider what information you need to give the other person. Can you just ask her to do something or do you need to explain why?

- Consider that the person might have other responsibilities and activities: be prepared to help.
- Be assertive (see Chapter 5), don't apologise for asking.
- Let the person know what feedback you want: should she tell you when it's done, or not?

Try an example:

Simi is an HCA and she has a reputation for not accepting delegation well. How can you ask her to stock dressing trolleys for the afternoon's leg ulcer clinic?

Here's the wrong way to ask:

'Simi, I know you don't like to stock the dressing trolleys for the clinic, but I can't do it all myself, so you have to do it, if you don't mind, OK?'

Try this instead:

1. **Approach her with respect:** 'Simi, I need an experienced HCA to stock the dressing trolleys; they need to be ready by 1.00 p.m., before the clinic starts, please.'
2. **Recognise that she might have other, conflicting, activities:** 'I know you are busy, if you need help getting your visits done so you can do this, let me know and I will see if I can get you some help.'
3. **Be polite:** 'Thank you Simi.'

Simi still might not stock the trolleys. If I were Simi's manager and knew that she might not get the task done, I would check to see if the trolleys were ready when there was still enough time to do it. I would then ask Simi to do it – now.

Simi might complain 'I still have patients to see!'. I would remind her that I offered to help, and later, after the clinic, I would go over her time management and see if I could help her plan other days a bit more effectively.

As a nurse, especially a newly qualified one, you need to walk a fine line: you have to be able to assert that you have the right to delegate and you have to make sure that the staff who work with you know that you will delegate fairly. Be a tyrant and they will make your life miserable. Be a pushover and they will make your life miserable. It's best for you, your team and – most importantly – your patients, for you to delegate appropriately because it maximises the time that you can do for your patients the things that only a nurse can do.

If you are struggling to delegate or organise your time, don't be hard on yourself: they are difficult skills. Speak to your manager or to a more experienced nurse: we all had to learn. Someday, someone will be coming to you.

Summary

- Nurses work to restore, promote, maintain and recover health, or to help people cope with health problems – allowing them to live (and die) with dignity, autonomy and independence.
- Nursing is both an art – with a requirement for technical proficiency and critical interpretation of situations and people – and a science – with a requirement for knowledge, judgement and decision making.
- With experience and practice, nurses develop intuition. Intuition is a hallmark of higher-level practice.
- Nurses work with very needy people: you have to have good boundaries. There are times you will need to walk a very fine line between boundaries – you need to make decisions for the right reasons and with the best judgement.
- Nurses are busy people – you cannot meet anyone's needs if you don't manage your time well and stress can result from not working 'smart'.
- Nurses need to organise the care their patients need: this doesn't mean doing everything yourself but you must only delegate when you are sure it's the right way to meet your individual patient's needs. Delegation is difficult but, with practice, it becomes easier.

References

Benner P E 2001 From novice to expert: excellence and power in clinical nursing management. Prentice Hall, London.
Henderson V 1966 The nature of nursing. Macmillan, New York.
Royal College of Nursing (RCN) 2003 Defining nursing. RCN, London.
Siviter B 2004 The student nurse handbook: a survival guide. Baillière Tindall, Edinburgh.

4 Research and evidence-based practice

- Research basics
- How to read research critically
- How to develop evidence-based practice
- Critical thinking
- Questioning practice
- Summary
- Reference

There are two key elements of research: understanding it and doing it.

> Research underpins my practice – it tells me what I need to do and how I need to do it (specialist nurse)

Before I start on research though, let's talk about hair dye. Let's say there is a commercial for hair dye, and it proclaims:

> Ninety per cent of customers say our hair dye is the best they have ever tried!

Sounds good, huh? But:

- What if they only asked 10 people?
- What if they only asked people who had never tried hair dye before?
- What if they only got paid for undertaking the survey if they replied in the positive?
- What if they asked people who didn't have hair?

OK, what if there was a commercial that said:

> Ninety per cent of our customers would come back and shop with us again!

That sounds really good! Until you find out that the options for the survey were:

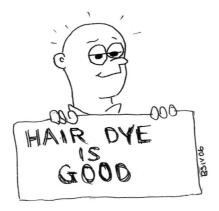

- Would you shop with us again if we gave you £10 off every purchase?
- Would you shop with us again if everyone else was more expensive?

I think you understand that it's not just what the research says but how it came to the conclusion. Let's try one that sounds a bit more nursey. Research says:

Eighty per cent of the people who take drug X return to work.

What if they were taking the drug to grow hair on their head – something that wouldn't impact work anyway?

RESEARCH BASICS

Research has to be relevant but it also has to have a certain quality and reporting standard. The thing with research is that you have to know how to decide which research is credible and which isn't.

Research can be very simple: it could be a literature review, where you find all the information about a particular topic. It can be somewhat complex: a wound-care audit across several teams. It can also be real academic research, using clinical trials and fancy statistics.

There are two different types of research and they tell us different kinds of things:

1. **Quantitative research:** is the more reliable kind and is used for things that need to be measurable. If the research is about the best

wound-care product, you would want to know which wounds healed the fastest and had the lowest level of infection.

2. **Qualitative research:** gives insight into thoughts, feelings and experiences. It's less important, for example when considering 'How do patients feel about larval therapy (maggots)?' to know that X% said they would never try it, than to know *why* they didn't want to try it. Then as a nurse, you could use the research to help you find a way to *your* patient.

Table 4.1

	Qualitative	Quantitative
Sample size	Usually small (10–20). Each person gives a lot of data	Usually large (100+). Each person gives a smaller, more specific amount of data
Reported using	Narration and excerpts; the data is usually narrative	Statistics, tables, charts; the data is measurable
Gathered through	Talking, interviewing, group discussions and open-ended questions	Questionnaires with set answers, reviews of data and demographical information, measurements
Replicable	Not specifically	Yes

Now let's look at an example:

Table 4.2

Example question:	Qualitative research	Quantitative research
What kinds of people become nurses?	Caring people, thoughtful people, people with strong backs, people who like dealing with other people, women	50% of nursing students are over the age of 30; 70% are women. Of 2000 people questioned, 42% said nurses were caring people*

*These stats are made up just to give an example.

See the difference?

Knowing the type of research lets you know what kind of data the research was based on and what kinds of evidence the research will give you. The first step in using research is being able to critically read it.

HOW TO READ RESEARCH CRITICALLY

This section is based on the section 'Reading research critically' in *The student nurse handbook* (Siviter 2004) – it really is the clearest guide for how to read research!

Research comes in different forms but each will have similar sections presented in it. In this section, I will explain the basic areas, and what kinds of questions you should be asking yourself as you read it.

> **Remember:** your goal is to determine if this research is appropriate for you to use as evidence to base your decisions and your practice on. You need to think critically!

When you are looking for research, the first thing you will see is the author's name, the title of the paper and its source (that is, the journal where it is published). These things start to tell you about the nature of the research.

Table 4.3

Section	What to think about	Ask yourself . . .
The author	You need to establish that the author is a credible person who has the background and education to write research/a paper of this type	Does the author have academic and/or research credentials? If you do a search for that author, what other kinds of papers and research come up? Where does the author work? What is his or her expertise?
Title	Should give you a small snapshot of what the research is about. The title should give a clear indication of the nature of the paper	What expectations does the title give you about the nature and content of the article? Is it clear and specific? Does it make sense? Go back to the title after you have read the paper and compare what you *thought* it meant before you read the paper. Is there a difference?

table continues

Section	What to think about	Ask yourself . . .
Source of the paper	You need to think about the kind of journal you found the research in. Some journals have a reputation for being very academic and reliable. Others might be seen as less academic and more 'fluffy'	Is this a credible journal (i.e. was there an article in it about how to cut the toenails of the Beast of Bodmin?) What is the journal's audience? Is it the journal of a particular group or organisation and could that present a bias?
Abstract and keywords	The abstract and keywords help you get a general idea of what the article is about. The keywords are listed to help you find the article when you search. If you want to find similar articles, search using the keywords	Read the abstract before you read the paper. After you read the paper, compare what the research said with what the abstract promised it would say. Did they match? Did the abstract leave out anything important?
The introduction	The introduction introduces the research question and sets the scene for what will come	Why did someone feel this was important to research? How and why is this relevant to nursing practice? Is the need for this research supported? Is the research question sensible? Is the research question something that is answerable? Is this the right kind of research for this kind of question?

Section	What to think about	Ask yourself . . .
Literature review	Doing a literature review is a real art. In the literature review, you will find other information and research available about the topic. To learn to do a thorough literature search, you will need to get a book about research	Is this new research a replication of old research? What has changed since any old research was done on this issue? Are the sources cited in the literature review accessible and credible? If there are other sources (which you would know about because you did a search), why haven't they been used? Is the literature review biased in any way? Are the other sources reliable and credible?
Sample	The sample explains who participated in the research, how they were found and why they were chosen. You need to look critically at the sample size and selection	Who was chosen to participate? Why? Were these appropriate sources? Is the method of choosing the sample appropriate? How long ago was this done? Has anything significant changed since then? Is confidentiality maintained? Is the sample size too big, or too small? Does the size and type of sample match the type of research being done?

table continues

Section	What to think about	Ask yourself . . .
Ethical issues	Are there any ethical considerations and how were they addressed? Research must be accurate but participants have a right to confidentiality	How did the researchers resolve ethical issues raised during or by the research, including protecting the confidentiality of the participants? Did the author get ethical approval for this work? Did participants give consent? How did the author find participants? Were there any special considerations for the participants? How is participants' confidentiality protected? Did the author have permission, from organisations, workplaces, etc., to do this research?
Data collection	How the data was collected? What method of collection was used and how did it work? This section should explain the tool that the researcher used. You should then look up that tool in a research text. This will give you the information you need to tell if the tool was used and applied properly	Is this an appropriate way to collect this data? Is the tool reliable? Is the tool used properly? Does the research type support the tool? For example, if this is quantitative research and a survey was used, did it really produce the right kind of data for that method?

Section	What to think about	Ask yourself . . .
Validity/reliability/ rigour	Validity and reliability are two terms used to discuss how credible quantitative data is. Qualitative researchers prove their data is accurate and correct by showing they rigorously used the correct methods and took every possible opportunity to remove any researcher bias	Does the data all make sense to you? If this is based on any other sources, are they credible sources? How has the reliability of the data been tested? Could this study be replicated with comparable results? Are there any assumptions being made?
Findings/discussion	This is where the researcher will tell you what the results of the study were. The researcher will refer back to statistics and information from the sections that have come before	Does it make sense? Is it useful? Does it match with the title and the abstract? How do these findings compare with the literature, both that in the literature review and that not included? Are the statistics reported accurately? Are findings reported in a way that appears biased? Do the tables, graphs and statistics actually tell you anything? Do the data collection methods and the data that is presented match? Compare the summary with the title, abstract and introduction. Does it all go together or does it seem like they are talking about different things?

table continues

Section	What to think about	Ask yourself . . .
Summary	The summary gives conclusions, which might include suggestions or recommendations. It might suggest areas for further study or highlight any particular problems or obstacles the researcher encountered. It should answer the research question	Does it make sense? Has the question been answered? Does it offer ideas for the way forward or to change/reinforce practice? Are there areas of future work that should be done as a result of this research?
Acknowledgements	This section tells you if the research was sponsored or done on behalf of anyone else	Did the sponsors or supporters have a vested interest in the outcome of the research?
References	References from the text of the article	Were any references left out? Does the author often reference himself or herself? Are these the sources that you would have used? How old are the sources? Are they outdated? Are they obscure, difficult to find sources?

Data collected for quantitative research are held to a very specific standard: the researcher must prove that the numbers and statistics being presented could be replicated in another study. In this way, the author proves that the information being presented is accurate and correct. Qualitative research doesn't have to prove it can be replicated – in fact, it is expected that qualitative research could not be specifically repeated.

If you are worried that the paper might be biased, get hold of a couple of the references cited in the paper and read through them. Does the way they present their data match the way they have been presented in your research?

When reading research, read the title, abstract, discussion and summary first. If the material is not relevant or useful to you, drop it. This will save you time over wading through paragraphs of methodology and design only to find out that the material doesn't really apply to you.

If you want to learn to *do* research, you can take courses in research that will help you. But, even if you never plan to research anything, it's essential in nursing that you can read research critically. Your ability to base your practice in evidence means you need to be able to tell good evidence from bad.

HOW TO DEVELOP EVIDENCE-BASED PRACTICE

What exactly *is* evidence-based practice?

Evidence-based practice (EBP) is the careful and considerate use of research and evidence in making decisions.

It requires practitioners to take applicable research and compare their own knowledge and skill to the recommendations from the research. Ultimately, it's up to individual clinicians to make the right decision about what should be done.

A huge part of EBP is the expertise of the individual practitioner. If you know something is the right thing, then that is what you should do. Let me give you an example:

Daisy has a leg ulcer, the last of half a dozen on her lower left leg. It's nearly healed. Research says that we should not use iodine at this stage of healing. But, we know from experience with the other wounds that her wounds heal faster if we keep using iodine.

Research says 'Don't use iodine'. The nurse decides to leave iodine on. Does that mean this isn't EBP?

No, because remember that EBP is the careful and considerate use of evidence in making decisions – it doesn't mean the evidence *makes* the decision – you're the nurse, that is what *you* do! You – as a nurse and experienced practitioner – need to decide what's best for your patient using all your available resources: research is only one of many resources. They key is that you actively think about what's best, not just assume and carry on without thinking.

If you just carry on then you will fall into bad habits and your practice will not be what it should be. Reflection (see Chapter 6) can help keep you aware of what you do; using evidence can help you make sure that what you do is the right thing.

Now, you can't keep up to date with everything – it's impossible – but you can do the best you can to keep up to date with things you do on a regular basis. Sharing good practice with other nurses and healthcare professionals can cut down on the amount of research you have to do on your own.

One way of integrating EBP into your nursing practice is to use the nursing process. Let's use an example:

> You are caring for a small child who is struggling to sleep. The mother asks if she should use lavender oil. Is there evidence?

Table 4.4

Nursing process	What is the question?	The answer
Assessment	What is the patient hoping the lavender oil will do?	The patient is hoping that the oil will help her child relax and get better sleep
Planning	Where can I look for research and evidence?	We have a consultant who does complementary therapy; do a search in the library There is a policy on complementary therapies
Intervention/ implementation	Is lavender oil effective for the patient's problem? Is there any information about how it should be used?	There is research that says lavender oil is helpful The research says a qualified aromatherapist is best suited to establish therapy The policy says we should refer to an aromatherapist if the patient hasn't had the treatment before
Evaluation	Looking at the evidence, is this something I can promote?	Yes, but I would like to have the child seen by a qualified aromatherapist

In the 'question' column, you should put the question that stage of the nursing process raises in relation to the issue at hand. In the 'answer' column, you put what you have found. If you actually write these out, you can put them in your personal professional portfolio (PPP; more about this in Chapter 10) as proof of your continuous professional development.

Let's look at one more:

> Maurice has had compression stockings in the past but it's been years since he has worn them. You haven't ever ordered compression hosiery and you don't know if they are appropriate now. His wife is asking if you will put them on.

Table 4.5

Nursing Process	What is the question?	The answer
Assessment	I don't know why we would use compression stockings, so I don't know whether or not my patient should use them now	I need to understand what stockings do, how someone is assessed to use them, and how they are used
Planning	Contact Tissue Viability Look for articles on compression hosiery	Tissue viability has a policy on compression stockings A current journal article outlines the steps in assessment
Intervention/ implementation	What does compression hosiery actually do? What are the uses and contraindications for its use? How do you assess for them?	Compression stockings help maintain venous circulation in the legs. You have to make sure that the person doesn't have arterial disease in the legs You assess by doing a Doppler, or by referring to a vascular surgeon You need special training to do the Doppler
Evaluation	Would it be appropriate for me to use these for my patient?	I can't do the assessment myself. I will refer the patient to Tissue Viability

You might want to add another level to the above: 'personal plan'. From what you have learned, is there more you want to know? Perhaps, in the second scenario, you have learned that you would like to become more familiar with assessment with a Doppler.

EBP, as shown by these examples, doesn't have to be about clinical trials and big fancy research papers. It can simply be the process through which you make certain that the decisions you make, and actions you take, are based on appropriate information and knowledge.

EBP isn't just about your response to specific situations. Many nursing journals offer research papers about current issues, with a section that allows you to reflect and consider how the research could impact your practice. Many NHS Trusts are developing care plans based on current evidence: you might be able to find a working group to which you can contribute.

Remember: the most important evidence is the well considered judgement of a competent, up-to-date nurse.

CRITICAL THINKING AND DECISION MAKING

Now that you have developed all these research skills, you need to use them in the clinical areas. You need to take what you have learned and decide what parts and how much of it apply in everyday life.

Critical thinking is the process of actively stepping back and looking at situations, analysing how things are done, thinking about different ways of doing things and trying in your head to apply different ways of doing things before you actually act.

You gather information through observation, practice, experience, learning and reflection, as well as through research and evidence. Using all the things you know, you critically appraise each situation and make a conscious decision about what you need to do.

Using critical thinking means bringing clarity, accuracy and fairness to everything you do; it means being able to hold your judgements up for examination and trust that you will be found to have used sound evidence and good reasoning.

To make sure of the ways in which they make decisions, doctors have developed a method of decision making called 'hypothetico-deductive reasoning'. In this method, they take everything they find – their physical assessment, the patient's notes, the lab. results – and they keep fine-tuning until they come up with a diagnosis. They keep going through everything that might be wrong and try to exclude it. It's as if they look at a picture of the patient and say 'It can't be a woman, the person in this picture has a moustache. They can't be old because they have no wrinkles. The person can't be in England because the Eiffel tower is in the background. Tah-dah! It's a French man!'. They use all the evidence they collect to prove what *isn't* wrong until the only thing left is what *is* wrong. That's why it's called *deductive* reasoning – you keep taking things away until only one thing is left.

Nurses tend to think differently. Because we are not diagnosing a problem, we tend to gather as much information as possible until we have built up a huge picture. We aren't interested in the one name of the problem, we want to know everything. Sometimes, perhaps, we want to know too much.

This is where critical reasoning and decision making are important. You need to be constantly thinking: 'Do I know enough?' 'Do I need to find out anything new?'. You have the tools at hand from the nursing process: assessment, planning, interventions and evaluation. You have the tools you gain from research and from evidence-based practice. But you need one more tool: awareness of when to *use* the research, information and processes you have learned.

There are two parts to critical thinking:

1. Having knowledge, skills and expertise.
2. Applying that knowledge, skill and expertise.

All the research in the world is useless unless you apply it. Ultimately, you have to decide if the research and evidence applies to your patients, their circumstances and their situation. Here is how you do this:

- How is the patient you have in front of you now the same or different from others?
- Are there any special or unique problems or situations?
- Is there anything that you don't know enough about? Are you confident that you have all the information you need?
- Do you need to involve anyone else?

You need to use a set of skills and practices to help you decide when and how to use the knowledge, skill and experience you have gained:

- Reflection.
- Experience: what happened before?
- Observation: what is happening now?
- Resources like evidence, policy, research, etc.
- Insight: looking for that one thing that others might miss.
- Confidence: that you have the 'big picture'.

- Challenge: you need to challenge assumptions.
- Open mindedness: you need to be willing to consider and accept new information.
- Communication: and the ability to work with others.
- You need, systematically, to gather and record information.

Let's look at an example:

Sue is a 55-year-old woman who has had a stroke. She is very angry, she refuses to work with the therapy staff and she demands that nursing staff get her up and moving. Because she is so upset, no one has actually sat down with her to ask her about why she is so angry.

The staff feel that her mood is being affected by the stroke so they decide to call in a psych. referral. But you talk to Sue and she tells you:

- That the physio keeps changing to a new person.
- That the physio made appointments and then didn't keep them.
- Sue feels the nursing staff are talking to her like she is a child.

Then you find out the following: Sue ran the customer service division of a large international company. She is a lifelong rambler who always walked to reduce her stress and her frustrations with work. Sue has a degree in – of all things – specialised physiotherapy!

Does this make you look at Sue differently? How can you use critical thinking with Sue?

Well, first you used it when you said to yourself 'I need to find out more'. Then you guided Sue through your interview in a way that helped you gather information. You now have evidence you need to bring back to other staff to help them help Sue.

Now you know that Sue is reacting to the therapists not because she is depressed but because she has specialist knowledge and skill and doesn't think it is being respected. She is having trouble building relationships with staff because they keep changing. She is a woman who is used to being in charge and isn't coping well with people who don't show up when they say they will. She wants to get up and walk because that's what she thinks will help her with her stress.

How can you help someone like Sue?

You have to think about the people who are also involved in her care. You have to consider the way in which other people work, if they will listen to you, if there are processes to go through – it's not always easy. You might need to use evidence such as the knowledge that Sue has a degree in physiotherapy to help you validate your belief that she is more knowledgeable than people might think. But ultimately, you have to decide, based on everything you know, how to go forward.

Is that enough? Perhaps.

That's the thing about critical thinking – you have to decide when enough is enough. Ask yourself 'Am I confident that the right things will happen if I leave this as it is? Or is anything missing?'. If something is missing, you need to keep going.

To be a critical thinker, you must:

- Have a foundation of knowledge skill and expertise on which you consistently build.
- Be open to new ways.
- Be willing to update yourself, constantly learning new things.
- Be willing to think about what you know and to challenge yourself.
- Work with others to solve complex problems.
- Systematically gather and share information.

Critical thinking and decision making is a skill like any other; it must be practised and developed if it is to work well. Don't use it only in 'big' situations – try using it as often as possible so that you get used to it. You will find that it becomes easy and commonplace.

QUESTIONING PRACTICE

It is difficult to see someone else do something and, feeling that lump in your stomach, to go forward and say 'I don't think you should have done that'. Even harder is going forward to a manager or supervisor and saying 'Nurse Debbie did something, and I'm not confident it was the right way'.

Sometimes you have to challenge policies, practices or even an organisation's entire strategy. In the real world, most nurses don't take these kinds of steps. Many sit back thinking 'Who am I to say some-thing? They probably know more than I do about it'.

Do they? There will be times when you know more than someone else and you have to be able to speak up. Some ways of doing this are easier than others. For example:

> Let's imagine that you see a nurse washing a patient. The patient had a soiled bottom and, to your surprise, the same cloth and water that was used to clean the bottom is used to clean the person's face.

You have a decision to make. Is it important enough to speak up about? It might be, but then again, it might not. Is it something you can live with if you ignore it? You have choices:

- You can ignore it.
- You can tell someone about it, but not tell the person.
- You can tell the person.
- You can gossip about the person.
- You can ask for help telling the person.

Let's look back at washing someone's face in water that was used to wash his or her bottom. Is this something that you can ignore? I don't know about you but although part of me would be thinking 'It's a one off', another part of me would be thinking 'Eeewww! That's disgusting! I can't let that happen.'

If you think you can ignore it, put yourself in the patient's place. Would you want someone to speak up if it were happening to you?

OK. So, you decide to speak up. You need to be careful. People have feelings and if you step on someone's feelings bad things can happen. Let's look at some ways you could address this particular issue:

1. (Screamed from one end of the ward to the other) 'Hey Marge! You can't wash people's face in bum water, what's wrong with you, girl?'
2. (To the patient) 'Make sure the nurse uses fresh water to wash your face, last time she used soiled water.'
3. (To Marge) 'Marge, I noticed that you washed Mrs Gascoyne's face with dirty water. We have a policy that you change the water, to make sure that the water you use to wash someone's face is clean . . .'
4. (To the team leader) 'I saw Marge wash Mrs Gascoyne's face in dirty water. Can you help me find a way to not let it happen again?'

And points for answer . . . 4!

You are a staff nurse, not the ward manager. You need to bring things like this to the team leader, ward manager, sister, etc. because they have the skill and knowledge to teach people how to do the right things. It will make it easier for you, and Marge, if you go to them.

Let's look at the possible effects of the other answers:

1. Marge decks you, loses all respect for you, runs screaming and crying from the building, and all the other patients recoil in terror whenever anyone comes near them. Not very helpful.
2. Mrs Gascoyne loses all respect for Marge, tells her family the nurse is washing her in dirty water, Marge's behaviour doesn't change and there is a written complaint. Again, not very helpful.
3. Marge asks you how come you think you know so much and starts gossiping behind your back, feeling intimidated because you questioned her on her practice.

The thing is, it's difficult to challenge people because they won't necessarily react the way you hope they will. As you build relationships on the ward, develop your communication and interpersonal skills and your empathy, you will gain insight into how to resolve problems like this one.

It is different if you are supervising someone. You might need to correct a student or an HCA. In most circumstances, if you are in authority over someone, you can't just ask someone else to manage that person for you although you can ask for help.

When you need to correct someone else, remember:

- Always preserve their dignity: speak in private and keep confidential things confidential (telling a manager is not breaching confidentiality).
- Ask for help if you don't know how or what to say (ask someone in higher authority).
- Say things that comfort, by giving the person benefit of the doubt: for example, 'Marge, it was really busy this morning and you washed 10 people, so I know you worked very hard and fast, but when you washed Mrs Gascoyne, you washed her face with dirty water. I know it's not something you would do on purpose, because you care, but I saw it and it's been bothering me . . .'
- Wrap it up: 'Marge, I'm not going to go any further with this because I know you know better; please be more careful and I will just drop this.'

The only time you can't offer to 'drop' something is when someone has been harmed as a result. You can't ignore a patient being abused, mistreated or harmed. You have a moral and legal obligation to tell someone. If it's hard for you to speak up, ask your manager for help in developing this useful, but difficult, skill.

Questioning practice is a logical follow-on from critical thinking because it is so closely related to the decisions you make on the ward or in other clinical environments. You must take seriously what others do. Sometimes you have to think 'It's just their way' and not get hung up on the fact that other people do things differently from you. But sometimes you will realise that the way they do things is wrong, and that they must be told that they should do things differently.

You need to be sure that, if you see someone doing something wrong, they are not causing harm or risk to that patient. If you see someone – anyone (even me: there, you have it in writing now!) doing something – you have an obligation to speak up.

A student once observed me doing an assessment of a patient's mental status. I asked the patient 'When did the Great War end?'. The patient was visibly confused for a minute; then she said '1908 – wait, 1918. Yes, 1918. You mean the First World War, don't you?'. And I smiled, and said 'Yes'. She smiled. The student said 'You confused her. You should have said "When was World War One".' I explained to the student that I wanted to see if the patient would think about it and, by her reaction, she showed me more about her ability to think and remember than if she had just said '1918'. I could see a look of understanding come over the student. She smiled, too; she understood. She never would have had that understanding if she hadn't had the courage to challenge. And now, when a student shadows me doing this kind of assessment, I take the time to explain that I might ask questions that appear to cause confusion but I do it intentionally. I learned from the incident, too.

Challenging practice means caring enough about patients to speak up for them and try to make sure that the right things are done. It's not about trying to make others look bad, foolish or incompetent and it's not personally blaming someone; it's about trying to ensure that we all do the best we can.

Summary

- There are many different kinds of research, and many different research designs, but they all have similar key elements.
- Qualitative research is subjective, about what people think and feel. Quantitative research measures things more concretely and is more objective.
- You need to understand the different elements of research in order to determine if that research is credible.
- You have to be critical about research so you can determine if the information it provides is credible, accurate and useful.
- Research is one of the foundations of evidence-based practice: your practice needs to be based on good evidence, and that

requires good quality research. Don't base your practice on poor research.

- Expertise is another element of evidence: an experienced nurse doesn't always need a research article to give her evidence for a decision – sometimes you just *know* what to do. This level of awareness requires insight and reflection.
- Evidence-based practice requires constant re-appraisal of skills and knowledge, and a willingness to see things from a different perspective. It requires that a nurse challenges herself and is willing to say 'The way I do that really isn't the best way'.
- You don't need to undertake research to understand it.
- Critical thinking depends on a set of skills as well as knowledge and experience.
- Decision making relies on critical thinking as well as evidence and knowledge.
- Nurses rely on gathering a lot of information to make decisions: a critical thinker is able to determine which information is most important.
- Challenging practice requires confidence, critical thinking and a desire to make sure things are done the right way.
- If you can't challenge practice on your own, you can get help from others who are more able than you, not just to challenge that particular area but to learn how to be more comfortable challenging in the future.

Reference

Siviter B 2004 The student nurse handbook: a survival guide. Baillière Tindall, Edinburgh.

5 The art of nursing practice

- Being an artist
- Assertiveness
- Assessment and nurse vision
- Communication
- Leadership
- Management
- Summary
- References and further reading

In Chapter 3 we talked about issues of managing your practice. In this chapter, we will talk about working with people.

The more I know people, the better I like my dog . . . (anonymous)

Working with people is one of the most challenging parts of being a nurse. In addition to the people for whom we care, we deal with many different professionals and personalities every day. If your nursing skills are exceptional but you can't work with others, you will never be a very effective nurse. Interpersonal skills are the avenue for delivering good nursing care; they are an art.

BEING AN ARTIST

Before we go into how to practise the art, we need to talk about *why* you need to practise the art. Anyone can measure blood pressure. Once, doctors thought that only they could, then nurses fought to do it, then we found out it wasn't a lot of fun so we let other people do it, and now – heaven forbid – we even let patients take their own blood pressures at home. What's that noise? It's not an earthquake, it's the uproar of thousands of nursing sisters – long deceased – spinning in their graves at the mere thought!

Once, we thought that being a nurse was about having the right uniform on. Wait, uhm . . . , sometimes we still think that. It's true, though, an artist needs protective clothing. But have you ever heard an art auctioneer say 'This painting was done by a man with a petrol blue tunic, so it is much more valuable than that old Rembrandt over there, painted by a man with a rip in his pocket!'.

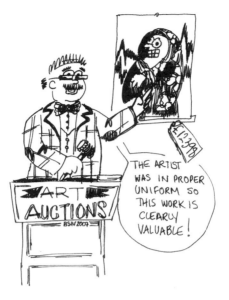

No. Being an artist is about more than just having the right clothing – it's also about having the right knowledge and skill for the job.

Being an artist also means doing something more with the bare elements. Have you ever done a painting by numbers? Does it look as good as the original painting on which it was based? No, because there are gaps, the colours don't blend into each other as smoothly, there are mistakes and places where things don't really fit.

That's why you have to be ready to be the kind of nurse who doesn't need to paint by the numbers. You need to be prepared to paint an original: one with no gaps.

Another part of being an artist is being proud of your work. When is the last time an artist said 'Oh, that old thing? Well, yes, you could buy it for £10 million but here, take it for nothing, it's not really very good...'. They don't say that; even school children want to be rewarded for their artwork: 'Mummy, either this goes on the fridge or I will never eat broccoli again'. As a nurse, you have every right to be proud of what you do. Anyone can paint by numbers, anyone can take a blood pressure, but you – you are a nurse, an artist, and you know how to provide nursing care that makes people feel better about themselves. You know how to prevent illness and injury; you know how to take the pain away.

Let me tell you something important: a lot of people out there will never make any difference in anyone's life, except for the kind of difference we all make – we brighten someone's day when we give them a gift or card; when someone loves us and we love them we make their world a place worth being in. But when you are a good nurse, you make a difference that no-one else can make.

As a nurse, you have a power that is nearly unimaginable. You can make it better. You can take the pain away, perhaps not always the physical pain but at least the emotional kind that comes from being lonely and afraid. You can soothe the fears and stop the panic. And you can do it in a way that looks easy. Some people can't be saved but you can still make it easier for them, through loving compassion and sincere sympathy. Use your skill and your knowledge to make a difference and some day, when a patient takes your hand and looks in your eyes, and says 'I'm glad *you* were *my* nurse . . .' you will know how important this wonderful profession really is.

You will never be the highest paid person in the world but how many people can take the pain away? And how many people can get the kind of satisfaction from their job that you can get from yours? If it ever stops giving you that satisfaction, stop and look, because you are going the wrong way. Don't keep going day after day being a nurse who doesn't want to be one – instead, be the kind of nurse who makes a difference, to your own life as well as to others.

From here, we will talk about certain types of skills and abilities. But I always want you to think about how you use them. Be an artist, not a nurse-by-the-numbers. Don't perform the skills, do *nursing* with the skills. Always look for the way to heal, to comfort, to fill the gaps and do the things that make the difference between a colouring book and a masterpiece.

You might be sitting there thinking 'I don't know if I can do that . . .' and you're going to expect me to say 'Of course you can!'. But I'm not going to do that: only you can decide what kind of nurse you want to be. Nurses are good at blaming everyone else – for saying it was short staffing, the doctors, the HCAs, the family – everyone else prevents us from doing things the right way except us. Look in the mirror and be honest with yourself. Acknowledge where you fail your patients but be just as willing to see where you excel. You will always do a little of both; even the worst nurse does excel sometimes. If you want to be the nurse artist – the nurse who makes a difference – then you need to plan and prepare. No artist became one without training. You have to learn the technical skills (the science) and become comfortable with the theories and beliefs, but only you can take the talent and turn your nursing into art.

Before you go any further, I want you to make a commitment, to yourself but on behalf of all of your patients, co-workers, doctors – everyone you will encounter as a nurse. I want you to make a promise to always do the best you can, to work as hard as you can and to be both proud of your work and unafraid of your failures. Yes – unafraid. Face them, thank them for giving you an opportunity to learn how to improve and then get moving and get better. And pride – be proud of what you do, let everyone who sees you say 'That one was born to be a nurse'. That's the kind of nurse who is an artist: the one who makes it look easy.

It helps to think about what kind of nurse you want to be: in the space below, reflect a moment before we go on. Which things do you feel are important in nursing?

- ☐ Assertiveness
- ☐ Communication
- ☐ Leadership
- ☐ Dealing with difficult people
- ☐ Reflection
- ☐ Understanding research
- ☐ Being accountable as a professional
- ☐ Tracking your accomplishments in PREP

All those things you ticked are the colours in your pallet. Grab your paintbrush: the lessons are about to begin:

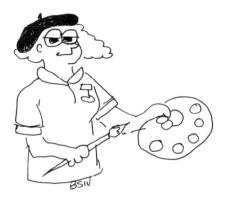

ASSERTIVENESS

When I speak to people about assertiveness, the most common comment is: 'I just can't *be* assertive!'. Try thinking of this image:

You are driving on the motorway. In front of you is a Robin Reliant, travelling at 37.4 miles per hour. What do you do?

1. Drive fast and go through it: it's only made of cardboard, after all.
2. Sulk, driving behind it at 37.3 miles per hour.
3. Keep charging at the bumper until the driver gets the hint and pulls over.
4. Assess that you can't stay here any longer, look in the rear-view mirror, determine when it's safe to overtake, put on your indicator, pull out into the middle lane and overtake.

A healthy person would do number 4 – assess the situation, decide the safest and best way forward, communicate with others and take the appropriate action. But, what happens next?

You've passed the Reliant, but . . . when you get home . . .

1. You take out an ad in every major newspaper so you can find the driver and apologise.
2. You rip up your driving licence so you don't have to overtake anyone, ever again.
3. You sell your car and move into a cave in remote Sicily, to spend the rest of your natural life doing penance.
4. You don't even think about it ever again.

It's number 4, again. But you knew that.

So, why can you be assertive when you are driving a dangerous, heavy, fast-moving piece of machinery but not when you are speaking to another person?

See, overtaking is really an assertive act. You recognise that something is presenting an obstacle and you take appropriate actions to go around. No hurt feelings, no recriminations.

If you think about the driver in the Reliant for a minute – how should he react?

1. He should make a note of your number plate, find out who you are and stalk you.
2. He should continue along his way, happily moving slowly towards his destination.
3. He should try to catch you and ram into you.

Gotcha – there's no number 4 this time!

But really, if he did anything but number 2, you would think he was a nutter. So why are you so afraid that people will react so badly to you if you stand up for yourself?

The way to make sure you get a good response from people when you assert yourself is to assert yourself *appropriately*. To do that, you have to think about what assertiveness is:

- Being respectful of the needs and feelings of others.
- Taking care of yourself in a healthy way.
- Protecting your rights, and the rights of others.
- Communicating honestly about your needs and feelings.
- Looking for solutions, not just complaining about problems.
- Not aggressive or bullying.
- Not manipulating.
- Not violent, angry or unreasonable.
- Not about shame, blame or being nasty.
- Not about getting even.
- Not about making others look or feel badly.

It requires practice and reflection to develop assertiveness skills. You need to understand what you are feeling and thinking to make sure that your assertiveness is healthy. As you reflect, you will see that other people react well when you confront them in respectful, kind ways.

The key here is that everyone – no matter who – is afraid at some level that they will be hurt, that someone will reject them or that they might be embarrassed about something. No one wants to be in a position where they look bad.

If your assertiveness can make sure that your needs are met, without the other person looking or feeling badly, then there is no need for that person to react badly to you. Some people still will; if they do, as long as you have done everything you can to be respectful and considerate, then it's not your fault or your problem. You can't make people behave the way they should. If you think you are so powerful that you can control the way people think and act, then you have a serious problem. Do the best you can to be the best you can be, and let other people worry about themselves.

If you don't assert yourself, you are putting yourself in an unhealthy situation. This is why you should be assertive even when it is scary:

- You will feel upset that you didn't stand up for yourself.
- If you let people take advantage of you, they will continue until you stand up to them or they grind you down.
- If you can't take care of yourself, you can't hope to take care of anyone else.

- Feeling used, disrespected, taken advantage of and powerless to speak up leads to stress and unhappiness.
- By asserting yourself, you could change things for the better for everyone.
- You have obligations, under the NMC *Code of professional conduct*, to challenge poor practice and to advance your own practice.
- You have an obligation, under the *Code of professional conduct*, to promote teamwork.

There are some times when assertiveness isn't a good idea: 'Excuse me, I know you are busy doing CPR, but you don't have an apron on and we are supposed to wear aprons if we are touching a patient's bed . . . '. If assertiveness isn't going to make things any better, don't go there.

How do you frame an assertive confrontation?

1. State the problem (remember, stick to objective explanations – no feelings, no blame, no shame).
2. State what you need and expect.
3. Show the shared value in getting a good resolution.
4. Know your limits, and think about what you will do if the person you are asserting yourself to won't work with you.

Towards the end of Chapter 3, I mentioned Simi, the HCA who was asked to set up a dressing trolley for a clinic. How could you assert yourself if she didn't do as you asked?

1. State the problem: 'Simi, the dressing trolley isn't ready and clinic is going to start soon.'
2. State what you need and expect: 'I asked you to have it ready, and it needs to be ready before clinic. Please do it now.'

Sometimes, you won't need to go any further – the shared value might not need to be put into words. However, if it does, in the next step (step 3) you are clearly telling Simi that preparation of the trolley is important for the clinic by:

- showing the shared value in getting a good resolution
- knowing your limits, and think about what you will do if the person you are asserting yourself to won't work with you.

So if after this the trolley still isn't set up, you will need to go to stage 4. Before you delegated this task to Simi, you should have thought ahead for what would happen if the task was not carried out. In this case, let's say you have to set up the trolley yourself.

You then have to go to Simi – and although it's not pleasant, you have to say something. You repeat steps 1 and 2:

'Simi, I asked you to prepare the dressing trolley. I told you that it needed to be done before clinic. I asked you in ample time and offered you help to get your other work done.'

Then you add step 3:

'We all work together here, and I expect that if you were not able to get this done, you would have spoken to me, so we could work together. You are a competent, experienced HCA and I rely on you to support our team.'

Then you add step 4:

'Simi, I am really disappointed in your work today. I'd like you to think about how we could have got through everything without the kinds of problem we have had today. Let's meet next week and I'll help you plan your day so you can get everything done.'

It's important that you do this in the right way:

- with neutral, non-threatening body language
- with an even, soft tone to your voice
- with appropriate eye contact
- in private.

No one likes to be scolded or humiliated. If you assert yourself in a calm, appropriate way it makes it much more difficult for the other person to react badly.

It's easier to handle the response you might get if you think about it in advance. In this case, you would need to know in advance what kinds of alternatives you were willing to accept. Planning for a 'win–win' scenario (where each side gets some benefit) is important in making a good assertive confrontation. Think: what are the end results that you would be willing to accept?

One important thing to remember when being assertive: don't be passive–aggressive.

Passive–aggressive behaviour is what happens when people are afraid of being angry, so they show their anger in a way that doesn't *look* angry. In the example above, you could have made a big dramatic show, complete with sulking, that you had to prepare the dressing trolley yourself. It won't do your relationship with Simi any good, you would feel worse and everyone would think you were a drama queen. After a few satisfying moments of self pity, you are worse off than you were before.

Second important point: don't manipulate or allow yourself to be manipulated.

People will react to confrontations in different ways, and they might act one way when really meaning something else. Perhaps Simi thought you wouldn't want to confront her, so she decided to ignore your directions. Or perhaps she was too afraid to speak up and tell you how busy she was. Clear, open and honest communication is essential to good working relationships.

If you know Simi struggles to get things done, perhaps giving her a task without helping her plan her work might have been a bit unfair. On the other hand, if Simi knows that no-one will say anything, no matter how little she gets done, then she might be manipulating you. Don't let yourself be manipulated or bullied. If you are being fair and reasonable, don't be afraid to raise your concerns at a higher level.

Third important point: this is about how *you* are feeling.

Start statements with 'I feel', 'I want' and 'I need', not 'you do' this or 'you make me' that. Don't put words in people's mouths. Don't say 'we all . . .' or 'everyone thinks . . .'. If you are the one asserting yourself then speak only for yourself unless you are there as a member of a group and the other members of the group have agreed that you speak for them. 'Simi, you never do what I ask you' isn't the same as 'Simi, I expected that you would get this done'.

Asserting yourself can be difficult, especially if you have been raised in a culture where it is not right to complain or it is wrong to speak up to people in authority. It takes practice. Find someone who is good at being assertive and ask him or her to help you. As you become more confident and experienced, it will become easier and more natural for you to be assertive.

Assertiveness is a powerful leadership trait and, as a nurse, it is essential to use assertiveness every day. You need it to delegate your work, to work with others and to challenge practice. If you are not being assertive, then you can't use the power and authority of your role to provide the best care for patients.

ASSESSMENT AND NURSE VISION

In this picture you see the usual, average patient area. What does it look like? Close your eyes and try to imagine every little detail, like where the call bell is, where the water jug goes, what the over-bed table looks like.

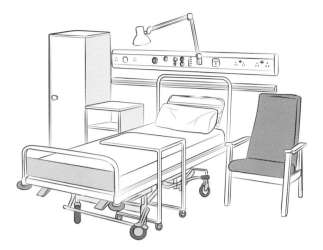

Imagine a patient in the bed. In a perfect world, how should it all go together? Where should it all be? How should the patient look? How is he or she dressed? How does he or she smell?

Now hold on to that image and, the next time you are at work, look at a patient. How is the ideal you have imagined different from the reality?

I want you to work hard on developing the 'ideal' patient environment in your head. Get every detail, and make it a picture you can't forget. Now, whenever you are at work, try to keep the environment your patient is in as close to the ideal as possible. It doesn't take an overwhelming amount of work. Just always think this way:

My patient should look better and feel better because I have been there.

Little things. If you work in a hospital, try to commit to the following:

- My patients will always have access to a way to call me for help, without having to reach or struggle.
- My patients will be dressed in an age-appropriate and dignified manner.
- My patients will be able to reach cold water to drink.
- My patients will look and smell clean and comfortable.

Imagine this:

> You are Gertie Parks. You are 87 years old and you have had a stroke. Three weeks ago you were independent and managing well; now, you are unable to speak or do much for yourself. The physio brings you a mirror; this is what you see:

- You are sat in a chair with your feet nearly touching the floor.
- You have facial hair.
- Your hair is in a top knot on your head, with a pink ribbon holding it up.
- You are wearing mismatched skirt and jumper. The jumper is soiled and the skirt leaves no imagination about what is under it as it is hiked up under your bottom in the chair. You are not wearing a bra.
- Your mouth has left-over food in it from breakfast.
- You need to use the loo but can't get anyone's attention, so the inevitable occurs.

When the physio comes back, she says 'Oh Gertie, you're drenched.' She yells out 'Can someone change Gertie so I can get her up?'. Two nurses whisk you to a loo and change you; they chat to each other but not to you. The only thing they say to you is 'Oh Gertie, I wish you had called us – this is a pain to change you up.' As if you enjoyed it.

The physio leaves without giving you any therapy, or any idea of when she will come back, because it took so long to get you ready. Your lunch arrives: creamed chicken, mashed potato and peas. Has anyone asked if you like chicken or peas? If they had they would know you certainly do not; they would also know you prefer coffee to tea. But, they shovel the food in, saltless and without giving you much chance to breathe in between bites. The mirror is still there. You watch the food drool from your chin to your jumper.

Then you see that you have no shoes on. Your old pointy toes dangle just above the floor, which has remnants of your lunch on it.

They leave you, as soon as you have eaten everything, with chicken stuck in your teeth and mash gumming up your dentures. And you need the loo again. Still no call light. You think to yourself 'Here I go again'.

What's wrong with this picture?

- Never call anyone by their first name unless they agree!
- Dress people in an age-appropriate manner. Top knots are for babies, not adults, and clothing should be suitable.
- People should wear socks and shoes or slippers. It's good for their feet and it's the way people appear in public.

- Give people choices about what they eat and how they eat it.
- You can find ways to listen to people even if they can't speak.
- Talk to your patients, not your colleagues, when you are caring for them. They are not objects.
- Clean people's teeth, ears, between their toes, clean their nails and trim them. No matter how many times it is said, it is *still* not true that you are not allowed to cut people's nails. It's an inconvenient task, but one that needs doing.
- Men have facial hair in our Western culture; women don't. If a female patient has facial hair, ask her (or her family) if she would like it removed.

Why have I gone through all this? Same reason we spoke about the environment. Keep in mind your image of what a patient should look and smell like and try to help your patients meet this. They should be sitting straight up in the chair or bed, appropriately and neatly dressed, clean and tidy in appearance, comfortable and ready to face the day ahead.

How would you feel about yourself if you were Gertie? How would you feel about the nurses and staff? Is that the way you want your patients to feel?

In summary:

- Have an ideal image of the environment in which you nurse patients; keep your patients' area in that state.
- Have an ideal image for your patients and help them be clean, appropriately dressed and attired, comfortable and dignified.
- Give people choice – about food, clothing, bath or shower – choice.
- Challenge others to do the same.
- Make sure each patient is better because you have been there.

Assessing people

An important part of nursing is being able to do for others what they would do for themselves if they had the ability, knowledge or skill. Without asking, how can you know:

- What your patients can do for themselves?
- What abilities your patients have?
- What knowledge your patients have?
- What skills your patients have?
- What your patients need from you?

Assessment is the cornerstone of nursing practice. It is the first step of the nursing process and it is the way you identify areas in which you will provide care and support. If your patients' nursing assessment fails them, then your care will fail them. Nursing assessment is the single most important part of the care you deliver because it is that on which all other care is based.

I can't teach you how to assess; you spent years in nurse education to do that. I can, however, help you remember to assess the right things in the right way, and help remind you should you forget why assessment is so important in the first place.

Get a good book on the Roper, Logan and Tierney model, take a course in physical assessment or shadow an experienced nurse and watch how she does it: however you choose to do it, you must assess patients well.

You also should assess them as soon as possible. Having a patient wait for assessment is like leaving your car in the garage for days before anyone looks at it – what's the point?

> Imagine this: you take your car in to the garage. It's been making a weird sound. When you come back to get it, they say 'We don't know what's wrong, so we changed the tyres and that should fix it.' You pay the bill and the same sound happens as you drive off. What do you think about that garage? You bring the car back and they do the same thing. Will you go back there again?

Assessment must be done as soon as the patient comes under your care, and it must be thorough, complete and consider the person as a whole person, not just as a patient. It must be legible, on the correct form, and signed and dated. Getting the information needed to complete the assessment requires tact, discretion and respect, good communication skills and the ability to listen not only to what people are saying but what they are not saying – you need to be aware when people leave information out and follow it up. For example, if you are assessing a married woman who never once mentions her husband, do you think perhaps there are problems there?

One of the biggest complaints I hear when I ask why assessments haven't been done is:

We didn't have time, it's been so busy!

Try this: have you ever considered assessing people while you are doing other things with them? For example:

> Today, you are Gertie's nurse. She hasn't had an incontinence assessment, mainly because she struggles to speak. While you are getting her washed and dressed, you chat with her about her

bladder and bowels. You have a giggle, a bit of a chat and at the end you have gathered all the information you need to complete the assessment. It's not rocket science – you just need to know what kinds of things to ask. You can find these things out by looking at the form.

The end result is that not only is Gertie's assessment done but she had a pleasant morning with you. You have made things better for having been there.

Perhaps you work in the community. There is another kind of assessment you need to know about: dashboard assessment. This is also useful for people who do home visits as part of their work.

When you enter the area in which your patient lives, look around. Is it clean? Well-maintained homes and gardens? Anything boarded up? Graffiti? Old cars? Trees? What kind of advertising? Are there bus shelters, shops, places to buy fresh food? You can tell a lot about someone by the neighbourhood they live in, and you can also tell if they are able to get their needs met.

Now imagine you are visiting Gertie at home (you already know her, so let's keep talking about her).

When you go to her home, you find there is a lot of broken glass on her street and there is nowhere to buy fresh food. If Gertie has no-one to bring her food, where does she get it? Does she feel safe? Is she safe?

What if you found tree-lined streets, a local shop and neighbourhood watch posters?

Don't judge people, but be aware of the special needs people have as a result of the area in which they live.

When I met Nancy Roper (who was as far from a quiet, reserved, delicate, fragile old lady as anyone you would ever find) she had a glass of red wine in one hand and she was pointing along with her lecture with the other. She was saying:

Assessment is about looking at a person as a whole person, engaged in a community, part of a social group, with needs, dependants and abilities . . .

Later, she said her biggest regret was that people saw her model as a checklist. 'It wasn't meant to be a paper exercise', she said. 'It was supposed to be a framework, a way to get people to think.'

Nancy was adamant that today's nurses fail their patients because they only want quick and easy answers. 'They want patients to present as little obstacle as possible', she said. Is that true?

When you assess someone, you need to make sure that you look at that person from all angles. You need to consider not just what is obvious and straightforward, but things that might be a bit more difficult to understand. It's not about completing forms, it's about using all your observation and communication skills to see who your patient really is, and what he or she needs from you.

COMMUNICATION

Everything you do as a nurse requires excellent communication skills. You deal with a wide range of people, with different cultures, languages and levels of understanding. You deal with people who are affected by emotional problems, physical problems, fear and worry – and those are just the consultants! All kidding aside, you have to deal with communication, some of it very difficult and very stressful, in a professional and appropriate way, every time.

There are three areas of communication:

1. verbal
2. non-verbal
3. written.

Chapter 9 deals with written communication/documentation. This chapter talks about how to communicate in a positive, non-threatening way.

You know, as nurses, we often don't communicate very well. We say a lot to our patients – but perhaps what we are saying isn't what we *should be* saying:

- We tell patients that they aren't important:
  - we interrupt patients when they talk to us
  - we make judgements and assumptions
  - when we are stressed and when we feel defensive we switch the discussion to things we can handle.
- We tell patients we are too busy for them:

- we focus on getting tasks done and see talking to patients as an interruption or a waste of time
- we talk to our colleagues as though the patient isn't really there.
- We tell patients that we are always right and we know what's best for them:
  - we don't always ask consent
  - we don't accept the patient's opinion if it conflicts with our own
  - we forget that everyone has a right to say 'No'
  - we explain things instead of just accepting how patients feel.

As an example:

> *Frank:* Nurse, my leg still hurts . . .
> *Nurse:* Well, what do you expect? Of course it does, it's got a gaping big wound in it . . . look, I'm a bit busy here and I need to get on, do you mind?
> *Frank:* Sorry, but just . . . nurse, my leg, can they save it?
> *Nurse:* Yeah, of course . . . I'll be back later, OK? You drink your tea.

What is Frank really trying to say? He's saying 'I'm afraid! Help!'. And the nurse is saying 'Go away, you are not top of my list of priorities'. How would it be if it went this way:

> *Frank:* Nurse, my leg still hurts . . .
> *Nurse:* (stops what she is doing) Frank, let me see (puts down what she is doing and comes to look). Oh Frank, it must be sore   do you want some pain medication?
> *Frank:* That would be good. You know, *I'm worried, my leg isn't healing . . .*
> *Nurse:* Frank, I know you are worried because your leg isn't healing but I don't think it's as bad as you think it is. Let me get you something for pain and we can talk about it. I'll make sure I mention to the doctor that you are worried, too, OK?

See the difference? In the second example the nurse does something called 'reflecting'. Look at the sentence printed in italic. The nurse took Frank's words and repeated them back to him. It shows that she was paying attention. It is a way of saying, 'tell me more'.

When you speak to someone, you have to be aware of what your body language is saying. Think about the statements below: match them with the body language in the second column.

Table 5.1

I love you	Arms crossed, hips cocked, foot tapping
I'm here to help you	Back turned, eyes focused elsewhere
You're important to me	Total lack of eye contact, ignoring the person
I am angry with you	Gentle touch on the arm, eye contact
You are not important to me	A smile with your face close to the other person's face
You are nothing	Arms open, hands out, eye contact, a smile

See how easy it is to match body language with the feelings? You could tell what some of those things meant without even looking at the words. Understanding and interpreting body language is essential. Before you could use words, you had to understand body language. You were two or three before you could even use basic verbal communication. Non-verbal communication is powerful and interpreted at an instinctive, basic level. You must be very careful to match what you say with how you look. If given the choice, people will believe the body language over the words every time.

KEY POINTS: BODY LANGUAGE

- Remember to make eye contact when you talk to people.
- Stop what you are doing.
- Move so that you are level with, or below the level of, the other person. Therapeutic talking needs both people to be at the same physical level. You can't show how compassionate you are if you are towering over the other person.
- Smile.
- Use your body's posture to show your attitude. A closed, turned-away posture is negative (arms cross, body turned to the side); an open, facing posture is positive (arms open, facing the other person, not defensive).

Did you realise how important body language is in our every-day interactions?

- We shake hands as a sign of friendship: we are showing we don't have a sword, club or other weapon in the hand. You have to be a friend for me to put my weapon down!
- We salute: again, to show that we are not raising a weapon. It's a sign of respect and subservience.
- We open our arms as a sign of friendship and comfort: we are welcoming someone in to our most vulnerable area – our torso. By exposing this area, we are showing we are no threat.
- We cross our arms to show anger or distaste: we close ourselves off 'I am not having any of what you are saying'.
- We divert our eyes when we aren't being honest: 'Look at me when you speak to me, I can tell you are lying by the look in your eyes!'. Mothers always say that, don't they! Well, they are right, as usual. Physiological changes from the stress of lying can change the size of the pupil. You *can* tell if someone is lying if you know what to look for in their eyes.
- We put a ring on the third finger of the left hand: 'I'm married'.
- A deep sigh when someone asks us a question: 'Oh brother, here we go again'.

Non-verbal signals are very important in our relationships and communication. As a nurse, you cannot allow feelings to creep into your body language. You must be aware of what you communicate, through words or otherwise. If we fail to communicate properly, patients won't feel safe and won't feel like they can really trust us.

So, why don't we communicate better with patients?

- We get very task oriented and talking to the patient gets in the way of getting 'real' work done.
- Sometimes, patients and families talk about things that we can't fix and it's scary for us.
- We might not like some people and we just don't want to be with them.
- Sometimes we are genuinely busy and really don't have time.
- Sometimes we just are too stressed or burned-out to care.
- Sometimes we are a bit lazy and sick of work, so we talk to friends to distract ourselves.

So how can we be better communicators?

- **Be honest:** 'Mr Brown, I can't talk to you right now – can we have some time in a little bit so I can really pay attention?' (Then make sure you *do* go back!).

- **Remember that you don't have to fix everything:** sometimes, patients just want to know that someone else understands how they feel.
- **Feelings and perceptions are personal, there is no right or wrong:** if a patient says, 'You are ignoring me!' you don't need to argue with them even if you are sure you are not ignoring them. It's OK if patients' feelings are different than yours. You don't have to be 'right': 'Mr Brown, I'm sorry that you feel I am ignoring you. How can I help you?'. Don't worry about explaining to the patient that you are right – that just makes it seem like you think it's important to make them feel like they were wrong.
- **A little sympathy goes a long way:** 'Mr Brown, I am sorry that this is taking so long, you must be very tired of all this.' OK, it's not your fault but when you are frustrated, doesn't it feel good to know that people understand?
- **Don't take it personally:** sometimes patients and families (or colleagues!) will act in ways that are very aggressive or unpleasant. Try to be understanding and patient. This doesn't mean you should be abused but try to see things from their point of view. Someone they love is sick; they are afraid; they might be in pain; they are not at their best. Don't argue or wind people up. They aren't really angry with you – they are angry about their circumstances.
- **Smile, touch, laugh, cry, be yourself (but see the note below):** it's usually OK to show a little of your feelings but you need to use good judgement. A friend once said 'You can always tell the best nurses – they are the ones who cry . . .'. What he meant was that nurses who show their feelings aren't cold or distant about the work they do. When people are ill, they want to be cared for by people, not machines. But remember to be careful that you are not using relationships with people at work to meet your needs; the patient always comes first. Be careful with humour – a well-intentioned joke could make it seem like you aren't taking a patient seriously. Use your judgement.

   Note: the real exception to this is when you are caring for people who have a mental illness or learning disability that could lead to the patient misinterpreting your intentions. You don't want to give the wrong message.
- **Don't treat patients as though they aren't there:** don't talk to your friend when you make Mr Brown's bed, talk to *him*. Don't chat away while taking his observations, ignoring him – it will hurt his feelings. He's stuck in the hospital, worried about getting better, and he hears you chatting about your big night out – how do you think it makes him feel? Take opportunities to communicate. Mrs Cecile, the lady who has had a stroke and is unconscious – talk to

her too. Perhaps, just perhaps, she can hear you. You might be the only person who speaks to that patient all day. Good nurses don't ignore patients.

- **Explain things when you do them:** how would you feel if you were in bed, couldn't see, couldn't talk, couldn't move, and all of a sudden someone was washing your genitals? Try to put yourself in the patient's place. Ask permission, even if the person is unconscious. 'Mr Tremayne, I'd like to give you a bath, OK?' Such a small thing can make such a difference.
- **Be polite:** say please, thank you, and excuse me. Address people by their surname (Mr, Mrs, Miss) until told otherwise. Introduce yourself. Ask permission. Don't assume Mr Tremayne will allow you to call him Vince; ask him if you can.
- **Don't force a patient to interrupt your conversation with your colleague:** as soon as a patient is near or approaches, make eye contact to let him or her know he or she has your full attention. Don't make the patient wait – you can talk to your friend anytime.
- **Talk is therapy just like medicine:** you don't need to be a professional counsellor to talk to patients. Just listen and be a friend (with good boundaries!).
- **Keep your body language open.**
- **Speak plainly:** 'Mrs Ewell, the contraindications of this therapy, including the potential for hyperacidosis of the upper gastrointestinal tract, which could result in hypermotility of said GI tract, outweigh the possible clinical benefit of the treatment; as a result, we are considering the efficacy of an alternative treatment.' Does anyone understand things when they are said that way? Why not just say: 'This medication can make you sick, so we are looking for something better to give you.' Don't call the patient's jaw a mandible; call it a jaw. Use big words to win at Scrabble: speak at the level you know the patient will understand. Make sure that patients and their families know they can stop and ask you what something means.

Using effective communication makes it easier for patients to trust you: this will improve the therapeutic quality of your relationship. But for those times when you can't sit and chat, you can still smile, nod and make eye contact. You have to use all the tools at your disposal to say 'I'm here because I care about *you*'.

As a nurse, there is yet another level of verbal and non-verbal communication. You will be working with some professionals who are accustomed to being treated in a particular manner.

Let me give you an example:

I telephoned a ward one day to enquire about a patient. 'Ward 17' was the way the phone was answered. I gave my name, and asked the person who she was. She replied 'Sister'. I asked 'Sister who?'. She said 'Ward Sister'. I was feeling a bit mischievous, so I said 'Did you parents really name you Ward? Or is your first name Sister?'. She sighed, deeply, and said, 'I am *the* Sister. Stop being such a problem, you know what I meant, and I have better things to do than entertain you . . . did you want something?'. To that I replied 'Well, I am *the* Consultant, and I'd like to speak to a nurse who has a name, please'. There was a very heavy silence on the phone. She then quietly said 'This is Lorraine (I'm using a pseudonym) speaking, I'm sorry, I didn't know who you were, Mrs Siviter, and its been a long day . . .'. The next time I went to visit her we had a chat about roles and titles, and we got to know each other as people. Now she calls me Beth, I call her Lor, and we get along well. Titles protect us from other people, but are our patients and colleagues really people we need that kind of protection from?

Other people are used to being ooh'd and aahh'd after. I know a consultant whose patient once said – after the consultant had spent a considerable amount of time trying to explain exactly how impressive his surgical skills had been in this particular case – 'Could you speak a little louder please?'. But no matter how loud he spoke, this very competent but somewhat arrogant consultant couldn't seem to be heard by the patient. Finally he asked 'Is there a reason you can't hear me?'. The patient replied 'Yes, the choir of angels singing your praises is drowning you out! Could I speak to someone without a halo please?'. The consultant's face turned red and he turned and fled from the room, hopefully to disband his heavenly fan club and allow less self-importance to get between him and his patient. There is nothing wrong with being proud of what you do as long as it doesn't get between you and your patient or work colleagues.

Titles and hierarchies, especially if they make people feel like they are more important than someone else, can be real obstacles to communication. Let me put a pin in a few hierarchal myths:

- Doctors are smarter/better/more important than nurses: nope, they just have more knowledge and experience in a particular area than you do. The doctors I know are puzzled by the reluctance of nurses to call them by their first names. Personally, I call the doctor 'Doctor So-and-so' when speaking in front of or to a patient but by his or her first name when speaking to them personally or when speaking with colleagues.

- Consultants are too important to be spoken to at all: nope. Consultants are in important *jobs* but that doesn't mean that they are a better, more important person than you or anyone else. Call them by their first name when speaking to them – it's easier, just as respectful and helps to break down barriers.
- Sister is more important than staff nurse: nope. The sister or charge nurse might have an important *job*, but they are still nurses, members of the overall healthcare team.
- HCA or students are not important at all: nope – no, No *NO*! There is *no-one* more important to the patient than the person who delivers hands-on care, or who is working to learn how to be a nurse, a physio, a doctor, etc. I found this out first hand: HCAs are usually well experienced in their post on that specific area and will often have more insight and intuition than any but the most senior nurse.
- Patients are more important that the rest of us; yes – this one *is* true. There is no one more important than the patient. Funny, we don't find it hard to call *them* by their first names, do we?

Finally, a note about the English language. Being from America, I have found that, despite being here for nearly 9 years, I still struggle with the English language. I'm not certain I can ever forgive the English for putting an 'o' at the beginning of esophagus. There is a theatre sister in Selly Oak who probably still thinks of me as an idiot because she sent me to get an OEsophagus tray and I couldn't find it because I looked in the 'E' section, causing the surgeon to wait (oh, dear!); esophagus made sense to me!

For other people, who might be from places where the language is even further from English than American is, the English language is challenging and difficult. Be patient with people who are trying. If they say something incorrectly, let them know in private. Don't just keep laughing at them every time they say 'I've got to set my fanny down, I'm so buggered!'. As soon as you stop laughing, I will explain that in American–English, that means to sit down as one is very tired, no reference to anyone's private bits or personal habits is intended.

But, if you can't understand what someone is saying, it is not being racist or biased to ask them to repeat, and even to go to your manager if there are real communication problems. As long as you are being honest, and not malicious, there shouldn't be a problem. It's important that you and your colleagues understand not just what you each say, but also what you each *mean*.

Communication is the foundation of everything we do: if you can't communicate, you are not going to be able to get anything done.

LEADERSHIP

Before getting into models, think back to your nurse education and remember Abraham Maslow. The 'hierarchy of needs' guy, pyramid, remember him? His theory suggests that until people's basic needs are met, they can't aspire to anything higher. At the bottom of the pyramid (the basic needs) are food, shelter and belonging; being confident and self-reliant are at the top. You probably learned that this was about patients – you keep them fed and watered and they get better – but there is more to it than that.

As a leader, you can't expect anyone to worry about improving their practice if the toilets are backed up and the lunch trolley hasn't arrived. Sometimes, good leadership means helping to solve the basic problems that people have and allowing their natural 'self-actualised' nurse to emerge, not because of anything you have done but because you prevented the problems from distracting them.

As a good leader, you will learn to get people to ask for help when they need it, to solve problems creatively, and you will remember Maslow's hierarchy: people can only reach higher levels of awareness when they don't have to worry about the plumbing, lunch and where they are going to sleep that night. This applies to nurses and other staff just as much as to patients.

Now that you understand the truth about leadership, let's go on to find out what kind of leader you might want to be.

Leadership models

There are a number of leadership models. Some of the most common are:

- **Transactional:** in this model, the followers give their loyalty because they get something in return. As long as the leader rewards (or punishes), they will continue to follow and do as the leader directs.
- **Transformational:** in this model, the leader inspires others to share in a vision, to think differently and to change things because they want to (there is a large section about transformational leadership at the end of this section).
- **Management-by-exception:** waiting for someone to make a mistake and then stepping in to correct the follower.

- **Impoverished/laissez-faire:** these leaders don't lead, they do as little as possible (more on this in the following section).
- **Authoritarian/autocratic:** these leaders like to be in charge, don't like to be questioned and expect that people will do as they are told (more on this in the following section).

I find the Blake and Mouton (1985) 'managerial grid' useful to help explain some aspects of leadership. In this grid, there are two concepts:

1. 'Concern for people' is plotted using the vertical axis, from 0 (impoverished) to 9 ('country club').
2. 'Concern for task' is along the horizontal axis, from 0 (impoverished) to 9 (authoritarian).

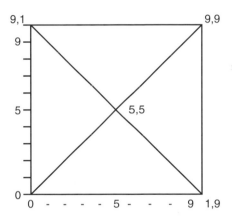

Along the horizontal axis, the focus is on completion of the task, success, perfection and doing what you are told. The higher the number, the greater the focus is. It's the first number in the expression.

On the vertical axis, the leader's focus is on relationships, belonging, shared decision making and communication. The higher the number, the greater the focus. It's the second number in the expression.

Most people would be balanced: they would fall at what I have called the 5,5 point. They can sometimes be bossy and authoritarian, at other times they are a bit wimpy but – overall – they care about people and they get the job done.

At the extremes (the 1,1, 1,9, 9,1 and 9,9 points) we find four different kinds of leadership:

- **Impoverished** (1,1): concerned about neither task nor people, this person simply doesn't care. He or she tells you what to do and then disappears. As a follower, you would doubt that this person under-stood what was really happening:

- pros: people are left alone to do what they want to do
- cons: there is no support and people feel leaderless.

- **Country club** (1,9): these leaders get along great with everyone, it's very social and people communicate well, but this is at the expense of the work and not a lot gets done. These leaders will use social events, chatting and strong interpersonal skills:
  - pros: it's fun and people feel good
  - cons: there are productivity problems, people aren't given much direction and, as a result, there can be a feeling that things are not very organised.

- **Authoritarian** (9,1): followers might not have any say and might not feel valued, but the work gets done. These leaders use sched-ules, policies, rules and blame:
  - pros: things are accomplished
  - cons: there isn't room for creativity, personal input or anyone who disagrees.

- **The team leader** (9,9) (for more, see the section 'Transformational leadership', below): these people inspire everyone to achieve. By motivating people to their best performance, the most amount of work gets done. People feel valued, and they value their personal contributions:
  - pros: people feel good, the work gets done
  - cons: can be dangerous if the leader's values are bad, because he or she is very charismatic.

Although the 'team leader' is the best leader of the extremes above, a wise and intuitive leader will use the others strategies when it is appro-priate. A strong team can survive a little autocracy when it's important; standing back can let new leaders emerge; sometimes the team needs to relax and let the work take a back seat. The key is that the leader can 'take the pulse' of the team and know what it needs to grow and progress.

In summary, Blake and Mouton (1985) look at leadership as a balance between the importance of interpersonal relationships, and the importance of getting the work done.

Where do you stand, on the Blake and Mouton grid?

Transformational leadership:

Another important leadership model is 'transformational leadership'. It has four key components:

- **Charisma:** the leader is someone people want to follow. The leader is confident, has vision and sets high standards.
- **Inspirational motivation:** the leader helps followers find meaning in the shared goals and vision.
- **Intellectual stimulation:** the leader helps followers to challenge and to think differently, and to look for creative solutions and new ideas.
- **Support for the follower:** the leader provides coaching, mentoring and opportunities for the followers to develop as people.

For transformational leadership to be 'authentic', the underpinning vision must be founded in a strong moral and ethical code.

Transformational leaders often use a combination of other leadership styles: they are good at getting people to 'buy in' to a vision by showing them the personal opportunities available. Giving incentives is an element of transactional leadership. Sometimes transformational leaders stand back and let others rise up – is this laissez-faire/impoverished leadership? Not necessarily: like the team leader in the Blake and Mouton model, the leader keeps a sense of what is happening and tries to give the team what it needs to progress.

So, what is leadership?

- Leadership is about taking risks, but those risks have to be taken with an awareness of policy, evidence and people's needs.
- Leadership isn't management but it considers the needs of managers.
- Leadership improves care and supports people in improving their ability to improve care.
- Leaders provoke people into acting and thinking differently.
- Leaders think creatively, solve problems laterally and see obstacles as inconveniences that, given time, can be overcome.
- Leaders change the culture and practices within an organisation, not just by their own work, but by the influence they exert over the organisation and the people in it.

How come some people lead and others don't?

- Some people have the drive and ambition that leads them to be a leader. Take Alexander the Great, from the moment he was born he was taught that he *must* be a leader. He was a proud, ambitious man – being a leader came naturally to him.
- Sometimes, people become leaders because there is no one to follow. In the Second World War, Audie Murphy (the most decorated American combat soldier of the war) became a hero and leader. When asked how he became a leader, he said 'Well, they kept

shooting, and we kept getting shot, and no-one knew what to do, so I did something. There weren't nobody left to lead, and if I didn't do something soon, there weren't gonna be no-one left to follow, neither'. It wasn't a big deal to him – he just logically saw a solution and acted.

- Some people become leaders because they want to make things different. They gain experience and skill, and start to look for ways to make a difference.
- Sometimes, sadly, people become leaders because they want power, control and authority.

People look for certain attributes when deciding whether or not to follow a leader:

- honesty
- trustworthiness
- honourable intentions
- having the right values and beliefs
- respectability
- someone they would like to be associated with
- having a vision
- being ethical and moral.

Some leaders are very effective: they can get people to follow them and accomplish work as a result. Some leaders – negative leaders – are not effective. They won't last long because people will stop following them. A leader who is more concerned with himself or herself than anyone or anything else won't last long because no one will trust them.

No one is 'born' a leader: it takes time to develop leadership. There are things you must do to lay the foundation for good leadership skills:

- Learn how to communicate effectively.
- Foster good relationships with other people.
- Reflect: know yourself, your strengths and weaknesses, and strive for continuous personal and professional development.
- Know what you are doing: if you want to be a leader, you have to have the skills and knowledge to back yourself up. If you can't walk the walk, don't try to talk the talk. People can smell a fake a mile away.
- Use critical reasoning and evidence-based practice: people come to leaders for advice, information and support. You have to be able to think clearly, make decisions, and come to sound judgements.
- Work to develop other people, so that they can advance, develop leadership and grow as persons and professionals.

What are some things you can do to demonstrate leadership?

- Help others with problem solving, planning and getting things done.
- Communicate effectively and honestly.
- Motivate people to get things done.
- Inspire people with your vision of how things should be.
- Keep your eye on what is most important; in nursing, this means putting the patient first, and keeping the patient's needs central to everything you do.
- Challenge: find things that need to be changed, and change it.
- Inspire others: have a philosophy or vision that others can understand and value.
- Teach and enable others: help others develop skill, knowledge and leadership qualities.
- Walk the walk: don't tell people what to do, show them.
- Share the glory: give credit to the team for achievements, and be willing to accept the 'credit' when things don't go so well.

One last note: if you think that being a leader means being powerful, you are right. There is a lot of power in having the approval of other people. But if you are going into nursing because you like having power, well, put this book down and start looking for a different career. As nurses, we are all equals with the same obligation to give the best care we are able to give at our level of education and experience. Just because you happen to be a leader doesn't make you *better* than anyone else.

When you see good leaders, you will know them. They are the people who inspire you, who give you confidence, and who role model the kind of nurse you want to be. Watch them and learn from them: that's the best way to learn leadership. And as you learn to be a leader, other people will be learning from you.

MANAGEMENT

As a leader (or a person aspiring to be a leader), you might think you need to get into management to use your leadership. But this is not the only place to be a leader: managers don't have to be leaders, just as leaders don't have to be managers.

Although there isn't enough room in this book to go into management in detail, I can get you started. Do you remember taking those horrible tests in school where they asked thing like:

If some zools are grebs, and some grebs are Zinks; are any Zinks zools?

Well, it will sound like that when I say 'Some managers are leaders, some leaders are managers, and some are only leaders or managers.'

First, management is different from leadership in that leadership is when people follow you because they want to and management is when they follow you because they have no choice. Management is organisation of tasks, people and resources. It requires using your skills to get tasks done, not just by you but by others. It then involves assessing those others, sharing that assessment, teaching others and being responsible when 'no-one' notices that you have run completely out of alcohol hand gel.

Managers have different philosophies. Some – genuinely – are born managers; they are organised, kind and considerate people who can act with confidence and use their professional knowledge to back-up their managerial decisions. Unfortunately, others see management as a way to score points and proceed further up in the organisation; others can't manage because they can't get their head around delegating things, or because they criticise people or make decisions on their own.

However, everybody can learn to be a manager. All the skills of management can be developed. Leadership, communication, assertiveness are all skills that are useful in any nursing. As a manager, additional skills such as report writing, research, audit, how to counsel and give bad news, how to coach, etc. are also important.

Think of the best manager you ever had: how did that person make you feel? What skills did the person have and how did he or she use them? All good managers have a few skills in common:

- They don't make you feel bad about yourself, even when you make mistakes.
- You naturally want to do things for them.
- You don't feel put down by them.
- You want to do what they want even when they won't find out what you did.
- You wouldn't consider backstabbing them.
- You care about them and know they feel the same.

Poor managers also have things in common:

- They often use threats and aggression to get people to do things.
- People fear them.
- People talk about them behind their back.
- People don't want to please them.
- You wish they would announce they have bought a house in New Zealand and plan to relocate soon.

A theory about management styles that I found really useful in helping me understand about managers is called 'X and Y' management. Each type of management is based on a number of assumptions:

- X managers believe that people are lazy, dislike work and will actively avoid work if given the chance. They believe that people like specific direction, want to be told what to do and don't really want any direct responsibility.
- Y managers believe that people need to be nurtured and taught how to develop, that they are worried about doing the right thing, worried about being good enough and need guidance and support to give them the confidence and knowledge to do the right things. They believe that workers want to be creative and need the chance to discover for themselves the way things should be done.

You might be thinking that X managers are jerks. But wait a minute, the Xs also believe that workers want clear, unambiguous directions: 'Do this *this* way and I will be happy and leave you alone.'

X managers work very well in some places– on large shop floors, on assembly lines – and there are some places that Y managers work well – in professional and academic arenas. Douglas McGregor discussed theory X and theory Y models in his 1960 book *The human side of enterprise*.

Are you an X or a Y worker? Do you need to be told or are you willing to work out creatively the best things to do?

In 1981, William Ouchi came up with a variant of the X and Y theory that combined American and Japanese management practices in a new theory Z. Z managers work in an environment where people expect:

- Long-term employment ('a job for life').
- Collective decision making, for example, working with staff and unions.
- Each individual to be accountable for his or her actions and decisions.
- Slow advancement – a worker might never reach management or supervisory status.
- Infrequent evaluation and appraisal.
- Informal control over employee actions, through policies rather than direct rule.
- Formal and explicit disciplinary measures.
- Specialised and specific career paths.
- Concern about the employee not just as an employee but as an individual.

The Z manager tries to combine both X and Y management styles, for different types of employees. Sounds a bit like the NHS, doesn't it?

How does this apply to you?

Is it important that the management of your organisation cares about your work–life balance? Or do you just want to show up, get your money and go home? Do you want to have each detail of your working life dictated to you or would you rather have some autonomy? It's a difficult balance for managers to do the right things for everyone, so they have to work hard to do the best they can for the entire organisation.

What does a good manager do for the organisation?

- Meets organisational goals in areas like finance, sickness and absence, inspections.
- Gets everyone up to the same minimum standard.
- Appraises people, helps them set goals, makes sure their needs are met in terms of annual leave days, scheduling, sickness, absence, etc.
- Makes sure the wards are staffed, the meals show up and someone is there to answer the telephone.
- Makes sure the bills are paid, the car park is maintained and that the vending machine has at least one tuna and sweet-corn sandwich in it (well, where I work that's important).

What does a good leader do?

- Inspires people to make good decisions.
- Makes people think 'I want to be like her' (or him).
- Encourages people to look at things in new ways.
- Helps people to take on new ideas and ways of working.
- Gets people to do the right things for the right reasons, not just because they are told to do them.
- Recognises people who work hard and try hard, who contribute to the joint effort.
- Helps people develop to meet a certain standard.

What do both do?

- Give structure to work.
- Give purpose and meaning to the everyday rituals of working.
- Give direction about the right and wrong things.
- Fix problems and give advice.
- Help maintain a certain standard.
- Recognise people who work hard and those who need to work a bit harder.

Being a manager isn't easy: you know how hard it is first hand. Is it easy to delegate tasks when people don't want the assignment you have given them? Is it easy to get people to work over Christmas and bank holidays? No.

Management is a huge topic. Bear in mind that everything you do as a nurse becomes management when you start to expect it of other people.

So how can you work leadership into your management?

- Instead of telling people what to do, explain why they need to do certain things.
- Give positive feedback when work is done well.
- Let people observe you, so they can learn first hand the way to do things.
- Be fair, and listen to feedback from those you manage.
- Learn about your own style and skills – as a manager, as a leader and as a worker – if you need a lot of motivation to be a good worker, you might not be the best person to be put in charge!

Summary
- Assertiveness isn't easy but it is an essential skill – and anyone can learn to be assertive.
- Assertiveness is not the same as aggression, bullying or making people feel badly.
- Being assertive is about getting your needs met, openly, honestly and without any hidden agenda.
- Communication is essential in nursing – it's the most basic and fundamental nursing skill.
- Communication can be the difference between things working well . . . or not working at all.
- Good communication requires that you focus on your patient and their needs.
- Leadership and management are different.
- Leadership is about being credible, having vision, and trying to make things the way you believe they should be.
- There are different kinds of leadership – some more effective than others in certain kinds of situations.
- There are negative leaders – people who have a way of making other people as miserable and unhappy as they are.
- Leaders aren't born – they develop, and everyone is capable of developing leadership skills.

- Management is about getting people to do those everyday things that we all must do to work together: show up, do our jobs and communicate about the basics. Leadership is about getting us to want to do these things better.
- Management theory and practices depend not just on the individuals but on the environment.
- A good manager makes things better; a bad manager can make things unbearable.

References and further reading

Bass B M 1990 From transactional to transformational leadership: learning to share the vision. Organizational Dynamics, Winter issue.

Bass B M 1998 Transformational leadership: industrial, military, and educational impact. Lawrence Erlbaum Associates, Mahwah, NJ.

Blake R R, Mouton J S 1985 The managerial grid III: the key to leadership excellence. Gulf Publishing, Houston, TX.

Kouzes J M, Posner, B Z 1987 The leadership challenge. Jossey-Bass, San Francisco.

McGregor D 1960 The human side of enterprise. McGraw-Hill Education, Columbus, OH.

Shamir B, House R J, Arthur M B 1993 The motivational effects of charismatic leaders: a self-concept based theory. Organizational Science 4 577–594.

6 Reflection

WHY REFLECTION IS SO IMPORTANT

When I finished my top-up degree, I didn't ever want to even think about reflection. I felt like it was pushed down my throat – reflect, reflect, reflect . . . so for the first couple months of my new post I didn't really think much about reflection. Then I noticed my standards were slipping – a student mentioned that I cut a lot of corners. I realised that my practice was going in the wrong direction and I needed to actively reflect on what I was doing. I'm back to regular reflection now. (qualified 2 years)

As a community staff nurse, I work alone most of the time. It helps me to share my reflections with other people, especially my District Nurse Sister. It helps me know that I do things the same way other people do, and that what I am thinking and feeling is normal! Sometimes when you work on your own you can get really critical of yourself. (qualified 1 year)

As a student nurse, you were expected to produce reflections to prove to your university tutors and your mentors that you were developing the insight and awareness you needed to become a nurse. As a qualified nurse, your focus changes slightly: reflection isn't really about proving to others – it's now about improving yourself because you *want* to.

As a nurse, you will make decisions without anyone really looking over your shoulder. This means that you have to rely on yourself and that inner voice to keep you doing the right things for the right reasons. It's not about what you actually do so much as *why* you do it. Reflective practice gives you the opportunity to think about *why* you make certain decisions and do certain things.

Why you do things will come from difference places within you. Some of the places come from your nursing experience and education:

- your nursing judgement
- your knowledge about nursing care
- your professional ethics
- your understanding of the NMC *Code of professional conduct*.

Some come from your life outside nursing:

- your general knowledge
- your personality
- your attitudes
- your emotions and emotional health
- your physical health
- your religion and culture.

Some of the reasons you do things will come from places you aren't really aware of:

- your memories of and experiences with people similar to your patient(s)
- past problems and hurt you have suffered
- your subconscious beliefs and needs
- your level of distraction and stress at the time of the interaction.

Everything you do is decided by elements from each one of these areas. Let's look at an example:

> Your friend asks you if you like her shirt. You make decisions at a conscious level – the style, the fit, the details. You know your friend is very style conscious and always works to look her best. You think about the question and what you want to reply.

But you also are also processing the encounter at an unconscious level. Your senses are gathering information without your active participation – what is your friend's posture? Odour? What is her facial expression? Your mind is looking through past experiences and old memories looking for situations that match this one.

You might reply to your friend 'It looks OK, I guess'. Not a very enthusiastic endorsement and certainly not the one your friend was hoping for. She asks: 'Why? What's wrong with it?'. You say you don't know: it's just something about the colour. You shrug. She pouts and walks away.

You might think: why don't I like that colour? It could take you some time to realise that the colour reminds you of someone that you dislike – and when you said you didn't like the colour, it was really that you didn't like someone who used to wear that colour. Perhaps if you didn't have a bias against the colour, you would have told your friend the shirt looked great and things would have gone very differently.

Your subconscious thoughts, memories and needs can all influence the way you behave and the decisions you make. Decisions strongly influenced by unconscious thinking might not be the best decision for your individual patients: most of the time, the things you think about in your subconscious are centred on you and getting your own needs met. As a nurse, you always have to put the patient's needs first. That's why you need to reflect: it's not enough to make decisions based on what you are consciously thinking; you need to be aware of less conscious things that might influence you. You can only do that if you take time to think about your decisions. Everything you do as a nurse must be, as much as possible, motivated by your nursing knowledge and skill.

Of course, with experience, you will develop nursing skills and intuition at a subconscious level. You can trust that part of your subconscious a bit more (there is more about intuition in Chapter 3) but you still have to be certain that you always do the right things for the right reasons.

That's why reflection is so important: it helps you look at the reasons you do things so you can identify those times and situations when you must work to override subconscious things. You might think that would be very difficult, but you have already done it: a nurse cleans up faeces and other unpleasant bodily fluids, but without a reaction. You have already learned to ignore the little voice that says 'I don't want to touch *that*!'. You also learned to ignore the subconscious reaction that would make your face turn into the 'oh that smells *bad*' look. You learned to override the instincts and subconscious reactions.

There is something else for which reflection is very valuable: research says that once you learn the basics of something, you go onto more complex things. That makes sense, right? But, once you go onto more complex things you stop paying attention to the basics to the same degree as you did before. This means that your practice in those basic, fundamental areas can start to slip. This concept is called 'entropy'.

Entropy is actually a concept in physics: it means that something will tend to increase in disorder unless something acts to prevent it. A good way of understanding this is to think of your house: if no one tidies up, it gets messier. That's entropy – it becomes increasingly disorganised and cluttered until someone decides to do something to put it back the way it belongs.

This can and will happen to your practice. Sometimes you might hear someone saying that they are being 'de-skilled' because they haven't done something in a long time – that's entropy: they have let those skills sit and as a result they don't work anymore. Reflection is a way of preventing that entropy from taking away the basic, fundamental skills you need in your nursing practice.

Reflection helps you to do the right things for the right reasons. To truly be effective, your reflection should not just be after the fact. With time and practice, you can use reflection to help you guide decisions as you make them. This is called *reflection in action*.

REFLECTION IN ACTION AND REFLECTION ON ACTION

Reflection on action

You will be familiar with reflection on action – it's the kind you practised in your nurse education. It's a formal, written process that uses one of those familiar frameworks, like those of Johns or Gibbs. Before going on to reflection in action, let's take a minute to review those models; you are probably already familiar with these:

Gibbs' model (1988)

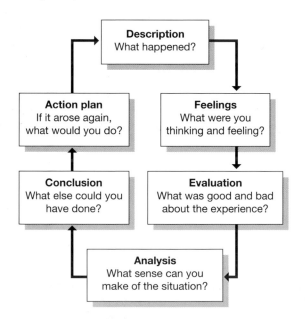

Johns' model (1994)

Johns' model of reflection uses categories with cues to help you think about and process your experiences:

- **Description:** write a description of the issue and highlight the areas you think are most important to think about. Identify the key people in the experience – yourself, your patient, other staff, etc.
- **Reflection:** think about what you were trying to do, why you did things and what the consequences were for those key people. How did you feel about this while it was happening? How did those key people feel? What did they do or say to let me know how they were feeling? How did I show how I was feeling?
- **Influencing factors:** ask yourself 'What internal and external factors influenced my decisions and actions?' 'What knowledge and skill did or should have influenced me?' 'What shouldn't have influenced me?'
- **Alternatives:** ask 'What could I have done differently?' 'What other choices could I have made' and 'What would have been the consequences of those choices?'
- **Learning:** ask 'How can I make sense of this experience, considering both the past and what I should do in the future?' 'How do I feel *now*?' 'Have I taken action to support myself, and others, as a result of this experience?' 'How have I changed?' 'Have others changed?' 'Is there anything I need to do as a result of this: take a course, apologise, read-up on something, etc.?'

In each of these models, you think about an event after it happened. That's what reflection on action is – sitting with your thoughts and experiences and sorting out what you did and what you would do next time.

But sometimes when you reflect you will find yourself thinking 'Why didn't I just do *this* instead of what I *actually* did?'. There are times that you need to work out what to do, not afterwards, but while you are doing something. This is called reflection *in* action.

Reflection in action

Atkins and Murphy (1994) is a good place for us to start thinking about reflection *in* action.

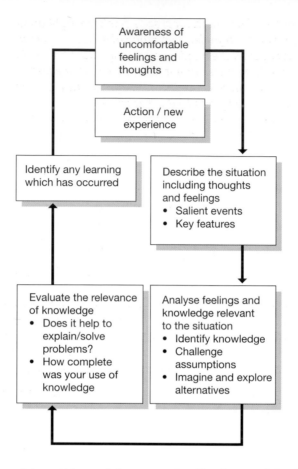

You can pick up this model at any point. That's one of the first points to remember about reflection in action:

As soon as you realise you need to think about something, stop and think about it.

I can hear you thinking 'How am I supposed to get anything done if I am always stopping?'. You have a point – but when I say stop, I don't mean to grab a cuppa and sit at the nurses' station. I mean to interrupt your train of thought and look at what you are thinking and feeling at that moment. As an example:

I visited Mrs Kaur to change the dressing on her left leg; the right one was only changed once a week and another community nurse had done it 2 days ago. I was packing up to go when I suddenly realised that I felt a little uncomfortable, but didn't know why. I almost pushed the feeling away but decided to

*think about it for a minute. I realised I didn't feel right about
the dressing on her right leg. I unwrapped it and checked it –
as soon as I opened the bandages a strong odour hit me. Mrs
Kaur sheepishly admitted that it really itched, so she had
shoved a knitting needle into the bandage to scratch. There
was a nasty infected wound. I don't know why I felt
uncomfortable, perhaps I had noticed the odour without
realising it, but I'm glad I listened to myself. (community
staff nurse)*

That's what I mean by stopping: pause and consider what you are
doing, by disengaging the 'automatic' nature of your actions. Reflection
in action can help you make sure that you are doing things in the right
way for the right reasons, and not just the complex or difficult things.
Sometimes, it's the basics that matter most. Using reflection in action
can help you make sure that your basic skills and care don't slip.

If you think your basic skills won't slip, think of this: statistically, the
basic, most common and most fundamental tasks erode most quickly.
Because you are so comfortable and confident about them, you stop
paying so much attention to them and they break down.

Reflection in action is a key part of critical thinking: if you train
yourself to also question, you are training yourself to always think
about what you are doing. That brings us to a second point:

Just because you have always done something a certain way doesn't
mean it is still the right way to do it.

When you do stop and review what you are doing, take time to
think if there is anything new that would influence your decision and
actions. Here's an example:

Amira is a community nurse. She goes into Mrs Bibi's home
once a week to wash her legs, assess them for any ulcers and to
reapply compression bandages. In the 18 months she has been
doing this she has left aqueous cream on the skin after she
finished washing.

Amira realises that she had read something about using
aqueous cream and leaving it on the skin. Before she was next
scheduled to visit Mrs Bibi, she spoke with the district nurse, who
hadn't heard anything about it. But Amira was sure there was
something – a little voice in her head encouraged her to not let
the matter drop. So she did a little research and she found
evidence that says aqueous cream should be washed off the skin,
not left on, as it can contribute to some skin conditions.

After talking to the district nurse, Amira could have just said 'OK' to herself and kept using the cream, but she didn't. The district nurse reviewed the evidence Amira found and changed not just Mrs Bibi's care plan but the care plans of a number of other patients as well.

The sense of discomfort or uneasiness you sometimes feel is a clue that there might be something there that you need to look into. By listening to your instincts and your intuition (more on this in Chapter 3) you advance in your knowledge and skill, and become a better nurse. When you get into the habit of reflecting it becomes something you do without even thinking about it, building your intuition. Because you are listening to yourself and reflecting on what you do, you should offer better care. But, how can you be sure? This brings us to a third point about reflection in action:

Reflection *in* action goes hand in hand with reflection *on* action.

Part of reflection in action is reflection on action. You can reflect on what you did and why, or just how it felt to listen to that little voice inside you: your nursing intuition. Perhaps you will want to reflect how you can go a step further and do more than just improve your own practice (you could use the notebook system suggested in the next section to do this). Perhaps you will see a way to improve things for a wider group of patients: you could change the world.

Who says it is wrong to want to change the world, after all? Would you want to be the kind of person who *didn't* want to change things for the better? Reflection can guide you to the kind of things that can make things *better*: for you, for your patients, maybe even for other people and their patients. What a powerful thing!

Now here's a bit of a challenge for you. Read the list below and answer – honestly – have you ever said or done any of these things? Then, come back in a few months, read the list again. The purpose of this isn't to make you feel badly, it's to help you remember about the basics and how easy they are to let slip.

Have you ever said:

- 'I'm too busy to help you, I'll come back later' and then not gone back?
- 'We don't have any toast' when you did, but couldn't be bothered to get it or make it?
- 'I didn't hear you' when you did, but really didn't want to hear the request or question?
- 'Can you ask someone else? I'm busy' when you weren't as busy as you made it sound?
- 'Let someone else worry about it, it's not my problem' when there really was something you could do?

Have you ever:

- Gone to the loo without washing your hands?
- Picked your nose and not washed your hands?
- Walked past a patient who needed help and conveniently not noticed?
- Walked past some litter or debris on the floor and not picked it up?
- Taken a longer break than that to which you were entitled?
- Documented that you did something when you hadn't?
- Promised that you wouldn't ever say or do any of these things?

I have some bad news for you: sit down, it's going to be hard to handle this.

Ready? You're human. You're not perfect. You can't do everything. See, I knew you would find this tough to swallow. As a nurse, you might think that you have to do it all – and then you get so stressed, tired and busy that you can't even get the basic things done. You need to know what you can do and what you can't. You need to know when and how to ask for help. And most of all, you need to know yourself and why you make the decisions and do the things you do. That's what reflection is really for, to guide you to being the best nurse you can be.

You are fighting a battle against entropy: if you lose, the patient will suffer.

DEVELOPING YOUR REFLECTION SKILLS: PRACTICE

This section is the outline for a notebook that you can use to work on developing your reflection skills. Get yourself a notebook and use this as a guideline.

Most practitioners, once they have been around a while, become rather adept at reflection – they just don't know it. One of the things that successful, busy people do is called reflection *in* action (RIN). The more basic thing that we all do is called reflection *on* action (RON), but RIN is a higher-level skill. Why? Because it is an attribute seen in people who are very self-aware, who are conscious of their feelings and actions, and who use this awareness and sensitivity to develop and grow.

Developing a sense of RIN will help you harness self-awareness and channel your growth in the right direction. It will also help you to bring plans and ideas to fruition. It does this through something called transformational perspective (TP). TP is the belief that, the better you know yourself, the more willing you are to learn and grow, the more easily you can adapt and develop better ways of solving problems and developing innovations.

Part 1: developing reflection on action

The first thing to do is read the text about reflection in this chapter. After you have done that, come back to this section – come back at the end of the day when you can have at least 25 minutes of uninterrupted time. Now:

- Think back on today: identify an event that either went really well or went less well than you had hoped.
- Try to write (in your notebook) what happened. Be descriptive. You might want to refer to the main part of Chapter 6 for some help if you are stuck.

Only continue with the next page after you are done. **Do not read ahead.**

Stop reading . . . go and write the story . . . **shoo – go!**

OK, now that you have written that out, identify another person in the scenario. Identify someone who was significant to the scenario. Think about why you have chosen this person.

Now, go back and re-write the scenario as if you were the other person. Try to imagine his or her thoughts and feelings, including how he or she might have thought and felt about you and your actions. Write this in your notebook.

Now ask answer the following questions (write your answers in your notebook):

- Was what happened today a fluke or is this the way things always happen for me? How and why?
- Is there something that the other person saw about me that I wasn't aware of? What is it?
- Did I choose a negative scenario – about something I did wrong? Am I more likely to notice something I did poorly than something I did well? Why?
- Is there something that happened in this incident that I would either like to do again or that I never want to have happen again? What is it?

Part 2: learning and growing

It's not enough just to know you did well or did poorly. You should take the chance to learn and grow.

- Think back to the thing you would like to or would not like to do again.
- Give it a name you can remember.

For example, if you are usually impatient in traffic and get a bit of road rage as a result (see the example in the section on assertiveness in Chapter 5), you might call this behaviour 'Traffic'.

- Now, go back to the text in this chapter about Johns' model of reflection (p. 125) and work through each of the categories.
- When you are done, think about how this behaviour comes about and what you might be able to do to influence the chances of that behaviour happening again.

To go back to the traffic example:

1. Description: I get stressed out and impatient with driving because I am in a rush and people go too slow.
2. Aesthetics: I get stressed because I see other people as being in my way.
3. Personal: I am feeling guilty that I am running so late and I am worried that I won't have enough time.
4. Ethics: I am not very respectful of the other people the way I act – swearing, giving needless hand signals, etc.
5. Empirical: I know traffic is heavy at the time I travel.
6. Reflection: it seems I am running late most of the time, and then I do tend to take it out on other people.

What's the answer to the problem? Poor time management. I am letting stress build up and vent in the wrong places. It's not the guy in the Robin Reliant making me late, it's me, and getting upset at him isn't doing me any good.

Do I want this to continue? No.
Plan:

- Travel 15 minutes earlier.
- As soon as I know I am getting upset, I will pull over and take three deep breaths.
- I will make an effort to listen to cheerful music in the car to help me be more positive.
- Reflect back in one week.

This next part will help you to follow the reflection with Answer, Continue, Plan. In this example, the answers are very short – yours will probably be longer.

- **Answer:** that which you have learned about yourself or the situation as a result of your reflection.
- **Continue:** your affirmation that you do or do not want to continue this course of action.
- **Plan:** i.e. what you are going to do about it. Your plan should be specific and creative whenever possible!

Next, choose one situation every day for the next week and reflect on it. Make sure you mix positive and negative scenarios. At the end of the next week, answer the following questions (write your answers in your notebook):

1. Am I more likely to notice good or bad things about myself? Why?
2. Are there similar things that pop up all the time?
3. Do I struggle with any one area of reflection (for example, ethics) that I really need to understand better? What is it?
4. Am I comfortable looking back at what I do? Why/why not?

Part 3: developing reflection in action

It doesn't take long to get used to RON. RIN takes real work.

Write the steps to the Atkins model onto an index card. Now, instead of waiting until the end of the day, choose at least one event as it is happening. Stop for a moment and quickly go through Atkins' model in your head as it is happening. In time, you will not need the card.

At the end of every day for the next week, reflect on what happened that day.

● Are there any aspects of reflection you are getting better at?

Now, a real challenge: start to reflect *before* you get into a situation. Think about the options, how you are feeling, etc. as you start to engage a problem or person. Reflect later on how that felt.

When you are able to reflect as instinctively and as naturally as you walk and talk, you will find that it gives you not only strength but a sense of purpose. You can use this sense of purpose to help change the environment in which you work so that it becomes stronger, more positive and more patient focused.

TRANSFORMING PRACTICE THROUGH REFLECTION

The way you practise is at the heart of everything you do as a nurse. Your decision making, your skills, the way you cope with problems – these things are the things that 'make' you a nurse.

Using reflection, you not only improve the way you cope with everyday things that happen but the way you do things overall. You have already seen how using reflection you can change the way you practise: reflecting on situations, you find better and better ways of doing things, you open your mind to new ways of working and you learn things that you might not have known before.

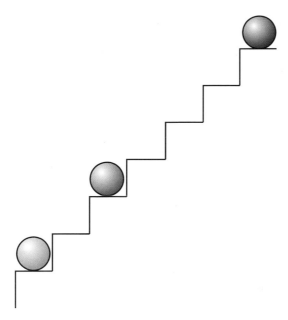

In this diagram you see an example taken from the theories raised by Patricia Benner in *From novice to expert*. In Benner's work, nurses start as a novice. They don't know what they should do and rely on others to tell them. They stand with their hands in their pockets and wait for direction because the world around them is confusing, chaotic and there is no way for them to see what they should do next. The dot at the bottom of the staircase represents the nurse – usually a student – at this level. The novice can look up and see other nurses on their journey in competence but doesn't know how to get to the higher stairs and so relies on others to tell them what to do.

The next steps are various degrees of experience. Benner lists them by name but the names aren't important – what matters is that you understand that your experience, decision making and skill all come in stages. In a minute I will explain how this relates to reflection.

In each of the following steps, the nurse realises what she must do without being told more often. She is able to look at the environment, at the patients, and say 'Oh, that needs to be done' without anyone pointing it out. She is starting to use the environment, rather than people, to tell her what needs to be done. The middle dot on the stairs shows a nurse in that stage of her development.

The final stage, as you might expect in a theory called 'From novice to expert' is expert. This level is unique: the expert nurse constantly uses her highly developed analytical skills to look for actions, to make decisions and to determine the best things to do. Her experience gives her benefit of a 'sixth sense', intuition about patients and their problems that sometimes makes others wonder how she could possibly know what she knows. The dot at the top of the ladder is that expert nurse. She can look back and see other nurses, and recognise where they are in their journeys because of the high degree of awareness she has about her own journey. These nurses often go into education or advanced practice because these are the places where the autonomy and decision making they have developed are most appreciated.

There are two things you need to know:

1. At every stage of your development you go through a mini 'staircase' of skills and awareness: you go from novice to expert and back to novice, again and again and again as you progress through various roles. You were a novice student, you became an expert student. You then became a novice nurse, and you now work on journeying through competency to become an expert.
2. You don't earn a place on the stairs and then stay there. You have to continue to work at it, because, in reality, the stairs are an escalator – they keep moving down and the world of science, health care and nursing is advancing – and if you don't make efforts to keep ahead then you go backwards. Nurses who rely on what they learned at university to keep them competent will soon lose competency, because the world changes.

This is why you need to continue to reflect, not just on everyday matters that might have caused you worry or distress but on things you might not have thought to reflect on.

The diagram below demonstrates a new way of thinking about everything you do, a way of using reflection to develop yourself as an expert practitioner. You can choose to stay at the level you are on, only ever looking at things in the context you find them (which is OK if you really do want to stay in the grade or at the level you are on) or, if you

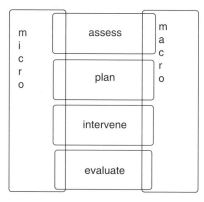

want to do more, you have to start to think more critically about the world in which you practise nursing.

The diagram introduces two new concepts into the nursing process – micro and macro:

- Micro: the smallest unit. This might be one patient or one ward; it is always the smallest unit of the unit at which you are looking.
- Macro: the largest unit. This might be a ward or a hospital. Again, it depends on what you are looking at.

Here is an example on how to use the diagram:

Ashe is a nurse in a busy hospital; he is the night supervisor. One night, a patient who should have called for help falls trying to get to the toilet on his own. Although the patient is fortunately unhurt, Ashe thinks about the problem, trying to work out how to prevent it occurring again. He sees that the patient's call light was out of reach, on the wall behind the bed. Looking around, he notices that most of the call lights have been left on the back board behind the bed, making it difficult for the patients in bed to reach them. He goes around his ward, making sure all his patients have their call light within reach.

He has a choice here: he can stop at his one ward (i.e. at the micro level) and be satisfied that all patients are now safely in possession of their call lights or he can move on to the macro level. He can, using his role as supervisor, check other wards. When he does this, he finds that many other patients don't have call lights either. He decides to ask other nurses to make sure the call lights are in place.

Following the nursing process, he assessed (checked to see if people were missing their call lights), he planned ('I will ask the other wards'), he followed through on his plan (the intervention) and now he can evaluate. His evaluation is a reflection: in it, he asks 'Have I done enough?'. That is the final step in the new type of reflection you can do to become more expert in your practice.

CONSIDERING EVERYTHING FROM MICRO TO MACRO, HAVE I DONE ENOUGH TO IMPROVE THIS SITUATION?

However, Ashe soon realises that because he didn't change the reason people left the call lights on the wall (he just moved the lights), the problem still exists. He didn't change the problem – he only changed a symptom of the problem.

He does an assessment of the situation: he looks at the problem and realises that patients move around a lot in the evening: they get their meal in the dining room, they might have visitors, they might go down to the shop or to the garden to sit with their family. Staff don't put the call lights out next to the patients because the patients aren't always there, so they put the lights neatly away on the wall. The problem is that when patients return, the call lights remain where the patients can't reach them.

Ashe has found it: he has identified the *real* problem he needs to work on. The problem is not that someone fell, it is that patients *must* walk on their own, without help, because they have no way of asking for help. If Ashe can fix this, he can help keep patients safe. He goes back to the nursing process:

Assessment: when patients return after the evening activities, staff might not be aware that the call lights have been placed out of reach.

Plan:

- Make staff aware of need to give patients the call lights.
- Check to make sure the lights are there.

Interventions:

- Raise staff awareness at hand-over and by putting posters in staff areas.
- Check to make sure lights are in place on rounds and ask other senior level staff to do the same. If they are not in place, remind the staff to put them in place.

Evaluation: Ashe plans to do an audit in a month to see if patients now have their call lights.

Ashe's behaviour demonstrates the difference between acting just on the one situation you are in (i.e. at the micro level) and using that situation to advance your awareness and your actions.

If Ashe had been a more junior member of staff, he might have stopped with the one patient who fell, reflecting on the problem that one patient experienced. Because he is more advanced, he viewed the problem as a symptom of a larger problem, and looked at the factors involved to try to find the larger underlying problem; and he found it.

Are you ready to ask yourself to look not just at the one patient but at the larger problems and issues? If so, you are ready to ask yourself:

Considering everything from micro to macro, have I done enough to improve this situation?

Don't worry if you can't answer this question, you probably won't have all the answers yet and it might be a while before you do. But at least try to move your questioning from the micro to macro level; always looking to see if something more could be done and using your assessment to gather information not just about the one problem but about the larger picture. This will help you to advance your practice.

Let's look at a couple of problems to help you get some practice:

> A patient falls trying to get through a door. You notice that the domestics leave buckets and mops by that door because their closet is next to it. The micro problem is that the patient fell. What might the larger problem be?

You will need to find out if the patient tripped over the buckets or the mops. Or did she slip on liquid on the floor from the mops? You might find that the fall is unrelated to the cleaning equipment; but, even so, is it safe to have those things there? You might feel that it's not your job to talk to the domestics but you might be able to at least raise your concerns.

> A visitor reports that their loved one hasn't had a bath and is feeling very grubby. You look in the notes and see that the patient is being washed daily but that there is no record of a bath. You ask a healthcare assistant to help the patient have a bath that evening.

Can you do more than this?

- How do you record whether patients like baths or showers?
- How do you record when a patient has a bath or shower?
- Is this the only patient with this problem or is it a bigger problem?

You might solve the problem for this one patient but is there a bigger problem to be solved? It might not be easy to solve but if you don't start to solve it, who will?

That is the real foundation of reflection: what can I do to make things better? In one type of reflection you look only at the one situation. In another kind, you look at the larger problem. Expert nurses look at the larger issues, using their experience, knowledge and relationships to not only solve the problems they find but the problems *causing* the problems they find.

Using advanced reflection and using reflection to change the way you look at problems and the environment in which you practise isn't easy. You will encounter resistance, because there are a lot of people on that escalator who are quite happy to be stuck at the bottom, having a peaceful life. If you are going to challenge, you need to be ready to take some guff. There is more about challenging practice in Chapter 4.

Summary

- Reflection is a necessary part of your life as a nurse: you use it to make sure you are doing the right things for the right reasons.
- Reflection is evidence of practice development and can be submitted as evidence to a hearing or as evidence of professional development for the knowledge and skills framework (KSF) or your post-registration education and practice (PREP) requirements.
- There are frameworks for reflection; they are all valid and any can be used.
- Advanced reflection means starting to reflect not after the fact but while you are doing something: reflecting *in* action not just *on* action.
- Advanced reflection also means looking not just at one problem, but the factors and problems that allowed that problem to exist.
- The elements of the nursing process – assess, plan, intervene and evaluate – can be used to help plan your steps to solve a problem.
- You can move forward and develop your skills, knowledge and experience or you can sit still. Sitting still, in a professional world as dynamic as health care, is the same as going backwards.
- Benner's 'Novice to expert' model reminds you that you have stages to go through to move forward. We all go through these and, when we change jobs or roles, we start as a novice in that particular area. You might have some advanced skills but you need to use reflection to help you identify the additional things you need to do to advance and become more proficient in your role.

A FINAL THOUGHT ABOUT REFLECTION

Everything is connected: it wasn't just the one problem, it was the system . . . it wasn't that the men weren't being fed, it was that there wasn't good food. It wasn't that the cook didn't make good food; it was that the good food didn't arrive. It didn't arrive not because it hadn't been ordered but because it couldn't get here. In order to feed the patients, I had to look many miles beyond our cook. It would be so much easier if things just happened as they should. (paraphrased from the diary of Florence Nightingale)

See, you are far from the first – or last – nurse to think that the world would be better if everyone just did what they should. You need to accept that reflection is necessary, in fact, important, and the key to making things better.

If you don't look at the situations you encounter and identify the problems that caused them, who will? Isn't that important for your patients?

References

Atkins S, Murphy K 1994 Reflective practice. Nursing Standard 8(39) 49–56.
Benner P 1984 From novice to expert: excellence and power in clinical nursing practice. Addison-Wesley, Menlo Park.
Gibbs G 1988 Learning by doing: a guide to teaching and learning methods. Further Education Unit, Oxford Brookes University, Oxford.
Johns C 1994 Guided reflection. In Palmer A, Burns S, Bulman C (eds) Reflective practice in nursing. Blackwell Science, Oxford, pp 110–130.

7 Mentorship

The student failed the placement because she failed to engage. She never once came to me to ask how she was doing, even when it was obvious she was failing. She objected to us using her a couple times as an HCA when we were short staffed, and after that I figured if she wasn't going to pitch in to help us, well, she could be on her own . . . (Staff nurse, during a disciplinary resulting from a complaint made by a student nurse who was failed but who alleged she had received inadequate mentorship)

WHAT DOES THE NMC SAY ABOUT MENTORS AND MENTORSHIP?

Nurses and midwives who take on the role of mentor must have current registration with the NMC. They will have completed at least twelve months full-time experience (or equivalent part-time). Mentors will require preparation for, and support in, their role. This should include access to a lecturer and/or practice educator as well as support from their line manager. (Standards for the preparation of teachers of nursing and midwifery: Nursing and Midwifery Council 2002)

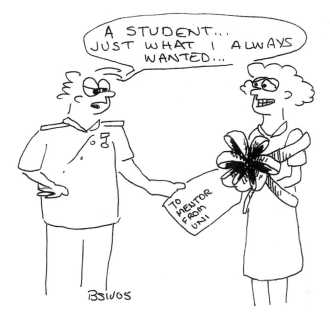

The reality is that new nurses are often asked to be 'assistant' or 'co-' mentors because there is a real shortage of available nurses. If you are asked to be a mentor, you must be prepared to offer support – you already know that part. But remember, you also have the right to receive support and preparation for the mentor role. Appendix 1 at the end of this chapter comprises a factsheet from the Nursing and Midwifery Council (NMC) about the preparation of mentors. It can guide you to ask for the development you need to be able to fulfil this crucial role as a qualified mentor.

The NMC also makes a strong statement, through research done on its behalf, that students must prove their competency in order to pass their clinical placements. In summary, the report found that:

- Students are passed on clinical placements even when mentors have doubts about their performance.
- 'Benefit of the doubt' or consideration for 'personal problems' led mentors to pass students who had not clearly demonstrated competence in the clinical area.
- Mentors should contact tutors/appropriate university staff, *in writing*, as soon as concerns are raised over a student's performance.
- Mentor preparation needs to be improved.

In response, the NMC put out a statement that said mentors need to be prepared to fail students who have not proven their competency, but that mentors are responsible for working with the student and with university staff to help students succeed in placement areas.

Basically, the NMC and the report highlight that mentors are the gatekeepers to professional practice and must only allow through those students who are able to live up to the clinical requirements and professional responsibilities of the role for which they are preparing. In addition, the report affirms that if the mentor must help the student become a competent practitioner, the mentor also needs support and preparation.

DEFINITIONS

Before you start, here are some definitions to the different words you may hear associated with mentorship.

- **Mentor:** a trusted counsellor and advisor, a role model, one who helps another to reach a level that they themselves have already reached.
- **Assessor:** one who measures and assures that an individual has reached a certain level based on certain criteria and expectations.
- **Preceptor:** a teacher or advisor, especially in an academic sense.
- **Supervisor:** one who has authority over another.

In reality, the words mentor, assessor, preceptor and supervisor are often used interchangeably. For the purposes of this chapter, I will use the word 'mentor' to identify the nurse who is expected to take primary responsibility for the development, assessment and support of a student nurse.

WHY MENTOR?

Student nurses spend roughly 50% of their course, about 2300 hours, on clinical placements. This is all the time they have to develop the basic skills, knowledge and nursing judgement they need for the foundation of their nursing career. They also need to learn our special language, our nursing hierarchies and the special tricks and tools experienced nurses have developed over time.

It can be difficult and stressful to be a mentor but few roles are more rewarding. Try to remember that mentorship is more than just showing a student how to document or give an injection. You are helping to mould that student into a *nurse*, a potential colleague and someone who will one day care for patients just as you do. This student might be *your* nurse in a few years. If you as a mentor don't invest in that student, you will fail not just that one individual but other nurses, patients and their families as well. Being a mentor is not just a huge responsibility to one student but to the entire health service and profession as well. The NMC recognises the importance of the mentorship role. The *Code of professional conduct* (NMC 2002) states:

> 6.4 You have a duty to facilitate students of nursing, midwifery and specialist community public health nursing and others to develop their competence.

There it is in black and white – it is your obligation under the NMC's *Code of professional conduct* to support students. If you find that you are not able to support students, either because you don't feel you have the skill or because you don't have the time or resources it is your obligation to speak up. This is also outlined by the NMC:

> 6.2 To practise competently, you must possess the knowledge, skills and abilities required for lawful, safe and effective practice without direct supervision. You must acknowledge the limits of your professional competence and only undertake practice and accept responsibilities for those activities in which you are competent.
> 6.3 If an aspect of practice is beyond your level of competence or outside your area of registration, you must obtain help and supervision from a competent practitioner until you and your employer consider that you have acquired the requisite knowledge and skill.

Although it is yet to occur at the time of writing this, there is always the possibility that a student nurse will raise an NMC complaint against a nurse who fails in his or her role as a mentor.

As a former student yourself, you know the frustration and stress that the lack of a good mentor brings. It's actually not that difficult to mentor – you already know the job and you care about nursing. All you need is to manage your time to include your student and the time they need. That *can* be a tall order at times, but it is possible. By knowing more about setting goals for your students, helping them plan their learning opportunities and understanding how people learn it will be easier. That these skills are also helpful when delivering patient education is a bonus that perhaps you hadn't considered!

We've established that it's a professional responsibility to teach, assess and support students. This support will come in many different forms:

- **Being a role model:** not actually having a student assigned to you but demonstrating good nursing through example.

- **Being a mentor:** having a student of your own who you will advise, teach and assess.
- **Being a co-mentor or associate mentor:** assisting another nurse in mentoring a student.
- **Writing:** you might consider supporting student nurses by writing for journals or even writing books that help students learn more about nursing.
- **Seminars/group teaching:** you could give an in-service for students in your clinical area, do a lecture at a university or give professional seminars geared to the student level at events like RCN Congress or a job fair sponsored by a nursing publication like the *Nursing Standard* or the *Nursing Times*.

Mentorship can be time consuming and challenging. After all, as a nurse you have many responsibilities and having a fledgling nurse following you around, asking questions and taking twice as long to do things as it would take you to do them alone, can be a real burden. So why bother?

- **The NMC *Code of professional conduct*:** as discussed above, you have an obligation to teach and support student nurses.
- **Someone mentored you:** remember how much a good mentor did for you as a student, and how stressful it was to deal with a difficult mentor.
- **You are a patient advocate:** adequately preparing tomorrow's nurses is essential to ensuring that patients continue to receive good care.
- **You are an ambassador for nursing and nursing practice:** by sharing your knowledge and skill, you are promoting and advancing good nursing practice.
- **You have an obligation to stay up to date:** students have a habit of challenging nurses and nursing practice, and this can help you reflect on your practice. Because they are actively in education, they might have new and more up-to-date information than you do. They also have 'fresh eyes' and their perspective might help you see your work area and your own practice differently.

Just a note: personally I have found that what I have received by supporting students has far outweighed the efforts I put into providing that support. Let me share part of a letter I received not too long ago from a student who had been in our team: 'After my last placement and all the grief I got, I was ready to give up, but you helped me realise where I was going wrong and now I know I'm going to be a good nurse . . .'. Think about that the next time you work three weekends in a row because you are short staffed. Potential nurses are a resource we can't afford to waste!

Trusts (and the NMC) require that you undertake preparation before mentoring students, but this preparation varies in duration and quality: some places offer a degree-level course, others simply offer a work-shop. And even though there are good intentions to make sure that mentors are prepared, the reality is that there are usually more students than there are mentors available to support them, so whether you are ready for it or not you *will* be mentoring students. This chapter isn't intended to replace formal preparation but it can certainly augment it and give you the basics while you are waiting to take formal training.

'Amnesia studentia' is an illness that can affect experienced staff. It is characterised by a marked inability to relate to the problems and experiences common to pre-registration nursing students. It is of concern because it is contagious . . .

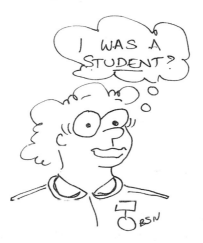

All kidding aside, it's important as a mentor to remember when you were a student, how you felt, how you were worried and how difficult it was when your mentor wasn't as supportive as you needed.

There are five important elements that you must consider when mentoring:

1. The student is a *person* who needs support, advice, compassion, inspiration, guidance and education in both theory and practice.
2. The student is an individual who will have unique needs and a personal learning style.
3. You have an obligation to make sure that the student is actually competent at his or her level, and to give fair and timely feedback about both positive and negative practices.

4. You must protect patients, make sure they consent to having a student involved in their care, and make certain that their care is never compromised: you are accountable for the actions of your student nurse.
5. You have certain documents and paperwork that must be completed (of course, this is nursing, what did you expect?).

In addition, you must remember that you and your student are part of a team of people and you have obligations to the team and the clinical environment.

BEING A MENTOR: WHERE DO YOU START?

First, get familiar with the paperwork and assessment documents used for student nurses in your area. Other mentors, placement educators/ placement facilitators, link tutors, etc. should all have these documents, and there should be a student resource folder in your clinical area.

Second, think about what your area can offer student nurses. Some common areas are:

- **Essential patient needs:** communication, hygiene, etc.
- **Documentation.**
- **Understanding different team roles and responsibilities.**
- **Processes:** how do lab results get to the clinical area? How are X-rays ordered? Where are the admission forms? Where do our patients come from?
- **The routine:** what do we do, and when do we do it?
- **Clinical skills:** learning how to carry out the daily skills needed to provide nursing care. Obs, nursing assessments, injections, etc.
- **Specialty:** what are the kinds of problems that your patients have, and how do nurses meet their special needs?

Some other areas that might not seem as obvious but are very important to students are:

- How to cope with the stresses of the clinical area.
- How to interact with other professionals and carers.
- How to solve problems creatively.
- How to delegate.
- What professional resources are important for a nurse in your specialist area: journals, texts, professional organisations, etc.

You might want to think about things that might not come up in discussion every day:

- **Ethics:** how do ethics factor in your practice in this area?
- **Holism:** are there areas of practice that might present a challenge to holistic, patient-centred care?
- **Law:** are there specific laws or legal issues that arise in this type of clinical area?
- **Professional issues:** what special professional issues are relevant to this area of practice?

Finally . . . knowing what you need to offer, think about how well the area supports students:

- Is there currently a morale problem in your clinical area? How will that affect your student?
- Is the area adequately staffed to allow you time to mentor?
- Is there currently such a staffing problem that you foresee the student being used to augment staffing?
- Are there teaching and learning resources?
- Are there any specific health and safety concerns for students?
- Do you have a ward philosophy?
- Does that philosophy include students?
- Is there a place for students to change into their uniform?
- Is there a secure place for students to store valuables?
- Where can they eat? Where can they park? Where is the bus stop?
- Is the role of students respected or are they seen as a burden or free HCAs?
- Is there anyone who has a negative attitude about nursing students?

If the ward environment is lacking in its ability to support students, you as a mentor (or potential mentor) should raise them with your ward management. Think back: would you have wanted to be a student on a ward like yours? If the answer is no, then improving the area for students will improve it for you and your colleagues as well: we are *all* students, no matter where we are in our career, aren't we?

Note: the NMC *Code of professional conduct* states that you have a *duty* to facilitate students' learning. This means highlighting possible problems in the clinical area that might obstruct their ability to learn, or yours to teach.

THE PROCESS OF LEARNING IN PRACTICE

The first thing to remember is that students will be placed in your clinical environment during different stages of their education. Newer students will probably need more help and guidance than more experienced students. It is important for you to balance your expectations against the student's experience and level. Because each student is an individual, don't just assume that a student at a particular stage in his or her course has a certain level of understanding or skill: you must discuss your expectations with the student.

Students will go through a number of phases during their time with you. Depending on their level and experience, some phases will go slower or faster. Try to see these phases as a continuum:

Phase 1: introduction
The student shows up, might or might not have experience, might or might not understand what kind of nursing goes on.

Student needs
- To be oriented to the environment.
- To have an initial interview (part of assessment process).
- A plan to get learning needs met.
- Reassurance about being wanted and welcome in the clinical area.

How to
Have a handout available. This will ensure that all students get the same information. Include: parking, shift times, contact numbers, location of necessary equipment/map of the clinical area, fire/health and safety information, where the off-duty area is located, general information about the type of clinical area and any essential terms the student must know. It is also a good idea to include a copy of the clinical area's philosophy.

Why is it important?
You know students need to know this stuff and it's easier to have it ready and hand it to them than it is to repeat it every time there is a new student. If students feel welcome and wanted, it will help their transition into the placement area. It would be useful for new staff as well.

Phase 2: shadowing
Student follows you (or other staff) around to get an idea what is going on.

Student needs
- To feel like he or she fits in with you, the team and the environment, and to build up enough confidence to engage in clinical tasks.

How to

Invite the student along as you do things. If the student offers to help, allow it, but don't ask. Some students take some time to get their bearings, others are comfortable pitching in: each is an individual. Having a student shadow gives you both time to get a feel for the other person: developing a relationship and communication will make things easier and more productive for both of you.

Why is it important?

You are accountable for the student's actions. By spending a little time getting to know the student, and making sure he or she understands what the clinical environment is about, you are protecting yourself, your patient and your student, and helping the student settle in to the clinical setting.

Phase 3: engagement

Student starts to ask questions and take on some tasks, under supervision and with support.

Student needs

- To be given appropriately sized chunks of work.
- To be assessed as competent before left to work independently.
- To be respected as a supernumerary.
- To be given opportunities to integrate theory into practice.

How to

- **Based on your student's level, make 'practice sandwiches':** you explain the task and do the first part. Allow students to do the part they *can* do and will understand easily, then you finish. As students become more advanced and more confident, the part they can do becomes bigger and the part you do becomes smaller.
- **Make certain students are competent:** discuss, then have the student observe you, then have the student do it while you explain, and finally have the student do it while you keep quiet and observe. After that, you can allow the student (of course, always considering law and policies) to have some independence. Encourage the student to ask questions and to be honest about their experience and abilities.
- **Document:** if students are engaging in the work of the placement area, make sure they reflect and look for opportunities to sign off competencies in their placement document. Also, remember that *you* can reflect on your mentorship!
- **Help students understand** and follow-through on all the paperwork and documentation related to the skills they are practising.

- **Feedback:** praise students if they are achieving well and raise concerns if they are not. Give students immediate feedback if there is a problem. It's difficult to say 'I don't think you are doing that very well' but you owe honesty to the student and to the patients that student will nurse. Waiting until a formal interview or assessment is neither fair nor productive.
- **Students are not there to replace staff:** they are supernumerary. This means that they are there in your clinical environment to get their needs met, not to meet the needs of your clinical area. Sometimes, what they need and what you need will overlap; sometimes, they won't. Remember to defend your students against being 'a pair of hands'. It's OK for them to help out as part of learning to work as a team but they must have support and opportunities to further their knowledge, skill and understanding.

Why is it important?
This is the bulk of your mentorship. This is where you teach, directly and by example, what it means to be a nurse. By helping students to engage in practice, you are helping them build actual physical nursing skills as well as helping them learn about themselves as nurses. As easy as it might seem to teach them to do something then leave them be as you get on with your own work, students need support throughout the engagement process if they are to understand not just *how* to do something, but *why* they are doing it and *what judgement* they need to exercise during the process.

Remember: nursing isn't just about competence in tasks. It's about competent judgement and decision making. Students need coaching and guidance to develop that nursing judgement.

Phase 4: assessment
Student and mentor discuss the student's progress and achievement. There are two levels of assessment. This section discusses the formal assessments made as part of the placement. You would use similar principles when informally assessing a student.

Student needs
- Documents from university.
- An appointment, scheduled in advance, for the midway and final assessments.
- Honest and fair feedback.
- An opportunity to give input and feedback about themselves, their work and the placement area, and about *you* as a mentor.

How to

- **Involve the student in the process:** don't take the document home and fill it in without the student being there. You need to discuss and involve the student in the process. Unless you have been with that student every minute of every day they have been on placement, you will need input from the student, and perhaps other staff as well, to assess fairly and accurately the student's achievements and progress.
- **Give the student dates and times:** in the initial interview, schedule the midway assessment and a possible final assessment date. The final assessment date needs to be flexible in case there are problems.
- **Quiet, private and confidential space:** assessment must be done in a 'safe' environment where the student can speak openly and freely. If there isn't anywhere available in the placement area, consider going for a break together and finding a quiet space.
- **Honest and fair feedback:** this is absolutely essential. If the student is doing well, say so, so he or she knows. Students often don't know how well they are doing and might be worried that they are not doing well at all! If they are doing something really well, praise them.
- **Failure:** if the student is failing, or if there are problems, this is not the place to bring it up for the first time . . . you need to raise problems as soon as they occur (more on this below). It's unfair to say in a midway assessment 'You haven't made a bed right since you got here . . .'. But if you have coached and counselled a student who still isn't getting it, then you can bring it up and make a plan with the student to improve performance. Students who are failing any aspect of the assessment at their midway performance need a plan to recover.
- **Setting goals:** the final part of the assessment is to set goals, or learning outcomes, for the placement or for further development. More on this in the next section.

Why is it important?

The whole goal of the placement is to have students develop skills, knowledge and competencies. As we say in nursing, 'If it's not written down, it never happened' and the same is true for students. Their assessment documents are like their final exam for your placement and should accurately reflect their achievement and progress. Completing their documentation also shows that you have fulfilled your role as mentor.

Learning styles

Before we get into planning and delivery education in the clinical environment, it's important to look at the way people learn. The way we learn is actually very basic – we learn by:

- doing
- observing
- hearing
- studying
- practising.

Some students will want to just dig in and start doing things, some will want to shadow you, some will want to talk about what you are doing and some will want to go away and read about it. Most will do all these things in different degrees, so your placement needs to offer learning in all these different ways. And every student needs to practise new skills and knowledge repeatedly for it to 'stick'. Doing something once is good, doing it a dozen times is better, but if a student gets stuck doing basics over and over it can actually cause *deterioration* in skill and knowledge. Having a student make beds every morning for his or her entire studenthood helps that student learn to automate the task and not think about it anymore, and once in automaton mode it can be difficult to get back into a learning mode. Students need varied experiences if they are to continue to learn. This means not just having students observe all the time, or do things on their own all the time. It means having balance. One way to provide that balance is to have a student follow a patient all the way through a certain experience, and to ask the student to research or prepare information on the experience. For example, a female patient is being catheterised:

> The student observes the assessment for the catheter after discussing the rationale for the catheter placement. The nurse takes the student to get the equipment, but instead of just putting it on the tray she asks the student to find and put the items on the tray for her. This allows the student to 'experience' what items are needed.
>
> The nurse asks the student about aseptic technique and briefly discusses the importance of sterility when placing a catheter. The nurse completes the catheterisation with the student as helper, and then the student is asked to go find information about catheter care and catheterisation. The student reviews the care plan and is asked to monitor the patient's intake and output for the rest of the shift. The student continues to follow the same patient on subsequent days. The mentor spends time discussing the experience at a later time when the student has had the opportunity to read up.

In this experience, the student was able to watch, listen, experience, study and then integrate what happened into a single clinical encounter. The chances are that this student will now have a solid understanding of catheters and catheter care, and will have much greater awareness of patient needs as a result.

Students should know what their learning styles and needs are, so it is good during the initial interview to raise the question 'How do you best learn?'. You can then help the student identify ways to make the best use of your placement.

PLACEMENT PLANS AND LEARNING OUTCOMES

Before getting into developing learning objectives, you need to think about the nursing process: assess, plan, implement/interventions, evaluation. This applies to students and their experience as well as any other part of nursing. You have already assessed your clinical area and have some idea what is on offer there. When you have your initial interview, you assess the students' needs by talking with them and by going through their documents to see what they are expected to achieve.

Now you will have an idea of what is expected of the student (through the assessment documents), awareness of what your clinical area can offer (through your own audit) and what the student needs from you (from your discussion and interview). This is your assessment. The next step is to plan and offer interventions to meet your and your student's goals.

You can help the student by setting up a learning contract (see Appendix 2 at the end of this chapter). This breaks learning into manageable steps, with time frames, and guides the student to not just learn the topic but to learn how to approach a new topic. It is very useful for newer students or for students who have very little experience in the area to be learned. More experienced students could prepare the contract themselves and have you review it.

Hint: photocopy learning contracts (with the student's consent and without their name on it, of course!) and save it for other students (or staff) to use.

It can save time and frustration if you develop specific learning resources, such as a database of learning contracts, for your clinical area that include a programme of study to meet common goals. Let me give you an example from an Ear, Nose and Throat placement I had at a wonderful hospital in the West Midlands. On my first day as a student I received a folder filled with information. The service area had reviewed the different resources it had available and put together a student pack that:

- described the service and the types of clinical services available for patients
- offered a schedule of learning opportunities
- included articles and patient information about common patient problems
- had a list of terminology and common abbreviations used in that area
- included a copy of the ward philosophy
- gave the names for all the staff and consultants
- contained contact details for charities and patient groups dedicated to certain illnesses or patient problems
- included a number of worksheets on common problems in that clinical area to help students improve assessment and critical thinking skills.

This gave me an opportunity to identify those areas and experiences most useful for my kind of learning. It was a wonderful placement area and even now I frequently use and reflect on the knowledge I gained there. (Thank you ENT ward! You know who you are!)

Even if you have a learning resource, you will still need to sit down with the student and go through the learning plan. Putting a learning plan together is actually very simple. The student will have some learning outcomes in his or her placement documentation. Commonly, it will be something like:

> 'Understand the correlation between physiological, psychological and sociocultural aspects of health and illness related to a specific episode of illness . . .' or something equally arcane.

It helps to translate the outcomes into English if they aren't already. For example, the line above says:

> Understand how patients' minds, bodies and everything else about them relates to what is happening to them right now. Think about how health, illness and lifestyle are all related.

Once you and the student understand what the goal is, you can break it down into learnable and assessable chunks. Let's look at a slightly more digestible goal as an example:

Learning outcome: demonstrate knowledge and practice of appropriate infection control.

The learning outcome is telling you what it wants the student to do. Let's take it apart. It is telling the student to:

- *Demonstrate*: the student is expected to model or show use of this knowledge and skill in practice. You will need to make sure you assess the student's clinical practice in this area.
- *Knowledge*: the student is expected to have a theoretical basis to the practice of this skill. You will need to assess the student's theoretical understanding of this area.
- *Practice of appropriate infection control*: the student needs to understand what infection control means in this clinical environment. You will need to make sure the student can relate his or her theory and practice to infection control. This means helping the student identify and understand policies and procedures relating to infection control.

Starting with the basics, you would then discuss infection control with the student to confirm that he or she has an understanding of what infection control *is*, and allow the student to express his or her understanding of its practice. This gives you a chance to see what the student really knows.

Sometimes, students will only need to fine-tune their knowledge and skill, but at other times you will need to establish a comprehensive plan. Using infection control as an example, you might want to establish the following as steps in learning:

- Find the infection control policy and read it.
- Identify tools used in infection control (aprons, gloves, hand gel, etc.) and discuss the method and rationale for their use.
- Identify potential ways infections are transmitted and how to minimise risk of transmission.
- Identify situations that commonly pose an infection control risk: toileting, dressing changes, etc.
- Identify appropriate ways of handling and disposing of infected or potentially hazardous materials and items.
- Practise good hand-washing technique.

You also might want to invite the student to teach patients about hand-washing or another aspect of infection control. Although not specifically in the learning outcome, you know that it's important and it is beneficial for the patient.

When you are working on the plan with your students, give them a chance to explain what they already know or have done, then you can figure out what else you need to give them. If they give you the right answers, challenge them a bit. For example:

> *Student:* Infection control means taking the steps necessary to prevent transmission of infection between people, and includes things like proper hand-washing, using the right technique when doing a dressing and taking care of things in the environment, such as cleaning up bedside tables, that could pose infection control hazards . . .
>
> *Nurse:* OK, that's good. What about how we handle things that might be infected, or pose a risk, like dirty dressings?

The student might satisfy you, for example by saying:

> *Student:* We put things that could be infected, or pose a risk, into the yellow 'hazardous waste' bags. Unless they could poke through the bag, like a needle, in which case they go into the sharps bins.

You can then let the student know that he or she has the basics you expect them to have, and then plan to monitor his or her practice:

> *Nurse:* Great! That's the right answer. I think you have the basics, but we'll work on your practice too . . .

If you then see the student *not* doing something, you need to tell him or her as soon as possible, while he or she is still able to think about what was being done wrong and why.

> *Nurse:* Amy, you just gave that lady a commode but I didn't see you wash your hands afterwards. Remember to always wash your hands . . .

You would then pay attention and see if the student had learned from your advice. If not, then you need to go back to the learning plan and establish goals to help the student really learn what you have identified as a deficit.

Sometimes, you will have a student who really shines. Using infection control as an example, the student comes to you with an idea.

> *Student:* It seems like the patients' families don't always understand why it's important to wash their hands. This is a surgical ward, and I think it might be good for them to understand about hand-washing. Can I put together an information sheet or poster on hand-washing? Maybe we can give it to patients and families when someone is admitted, to help them remember . . .

Perhaps your clinical area has these posters already and you really don't think this is necessary. Don't immediately react and say 'no'. Ask more about what the student would like to do and, unless it really is completely unnecessary, give him or her some time to try. By doing this, you might come up with something that really benefits your patients and your clinical environment, and you will certainly help the student learn to innovate and problem solve. The worst that will happen is that you won't use what the student has done: that doesn't mean it wasn't useful for him or her to try.

To summarise about learning outcomes and planning:

- Break goals into manageable, understandable, assessable chunks.
- Always help students relate theory to practice.
- Give students a chance to read, research and look at policies, protocols, etc.
- Help students recognise opportunities in your clinical area to practise their skills and increase their knowledge.
- Be concrete and specific when telling the student what you want.
- Allow students to explain what they already know and what they think they need.
- Let students know right away if there is a problem.
- Give students positive feedback if they are doing well.
- Allow students to develop creative ideas and to innovate when possible.
- If a student raises a valid concern or complaint about the clinical area, investigate. If the student is right, involve him or her in improving the situation. Document in the assessment document that the student took a proactive approach to his or her practice.

A NOTE ON FAILURE

You must fail a student if that person is not safe or not competent. However, before it gets to the final 'You've failed' stage, you need to make sure that you have given the student every opportunity to achieve and be successful.

You must give students timely and immediate feedback if they make a mistake, and give them a chance to overcome any gaps in knowledge or skill. Don't wait until the assessment interview: take them aside right away.

Also, don't just take a colleague's word that a student is or isn't achieving: you are the mentor, you need to observe and discuss with the student yourself to determine how well he or she is doing.

Your job as a mentor is twofold: to teach the student and to protect patients from bad practice. If you don't tell students when they aren't doing well, you are not fulfilling either role!

If you feel like you can't confront a student, then immediately ask for help from the practice placement manager or from your own manager.

Equally, if you don't tell students when they are doing well then they won't know for sure that they are succeeding.

COMMON WORRIES EXPRESSED BY MENTORS

- The student doesn't show up for the placement, is off sick for extended periods or doesn't engage in the placement area.
- The student is not behaving appropriately (in dress, manner, appearance, etc.).
- The student doesn't have a clue what to do or why.
- The student isn't safe to practise.
- The student is doing *dumb* things.
- The student is following you around like a motherless puppy and is driving you mad.
- The student is arrogant and know-it-all-ish.
- You have explained/demonstrated the same thing umpteen times and the student still doesn't get it.

OK, the solutions to all of these worries will be different in each circumstance and for each individual, but the way you need to start solving them lies in communication.

As soon as you realise there is a problem, *you* need to reflect on the situation and on your reaction to it. Before you bring it to the student, get it clear in your own mind. When you discuss things, give concrete examples, and try to offer them objectively.

Give the student a chance to put across his or her side of the story. If you can't listen objectively, get someone else involved.

If it's a serious issue like safety, get support from the university and/or your clinical area's placement manager.

After reflecting and discussing with the student, make a plan to move forward. Make sure you let the student know you are still willing to support him or her and that his or her mistakes are not going to be held against them if they improve.

Some worries mentors have are less to do with the students than with themselves:

- The student is asking you questions and you don't have a clue what the answers are.
- The student asks too many questions or challenges things in the area and colleagues are giving you grief as a result.
- You are short staffed and don't have time to cope with a student.

Again, reflect. Think about the NMC *Code of professional conduct*. Think back to your nursing student days. Think about your personal and professional ethics. What is the right thing to do?

Sometimes, your student will help *you* learn or will provoke a change in your clinical area. If so, see it as a positive and productive process. If other staff are giving you or your student grief because the student is asking valid questions or appropriately challenging practice, seek support from your clinical area's management. Students must know they can ask questions and challenge practice: it is an essential part of their development.

If your area is too short staffed to support the student, then think about creative ways to meet the student's needs. A note here: *this doesn't mean making the student into an HCA for the day*. It means helping find meaningful tasks, which might or might not be carried out on your clinical area. Perhaps asking the student to take some time in the library to research something until a 'safe' time to return is better than having the student feel used and abused. You also have a professional obligation to raise your concerns with your management if there isn't enough time or staff to support students.

Summary
- You have a professional responsibility to facilitate learning for students.
- If you feel you aren't able to support students, for whatever reason, you have to raise your concerns with your management.

- The process of mentoring is based on the nursing process: assess, plan, implement/interventions, evaluation.
- Students will go through a number of stages during the placement: the goal is to get them to engage in practice, both so you can assess them and so they can have experience in developing and demonstrating nursing knowledge and skill.
- Make sure students have clear, specific goals for their placement.
- Make sure students are involved in setting their goals.
- Give timely, appropriate feedback when things go well and when they go badly.
- If a student fails, then don't pass him or her but make sure you have done everything you can to help that person succeed.
- Reflect on situations and on your role as a mentor.
- It's hard enough being a student: don't make it any more difficult for the students than it has to be. Welcome them, teach them, support them and protect them when necessary.

References

Nursing and Midwifery Council (NMC) 2002 Code of professional conduct. NMC, London.
Nursing and Midwifery Council (NMC) 2002 Standards for the preparation of teachers of nursing and midwifery. NMC, London.

Useful reading

The following are some books you might find useful: these books are in plain English, written by nurses who have spent time in clinical practice and many of whom have been actively involved as advocates for student nurses:

Duffy K 2004 Failing students. Glasgow Caledonian University, Glasgow.
Hinchcliff S, Eaton A, Howard S, Thomson S 2004 The practitioner as teacher. Churchill Livingstone, Edinburgh.
Howard S, Eaton A 2003 The practitioner as assessor. Baillière Tindall, Edinburgh.
Oliver E, Endersby C 1994 Teaching and assessing nurses: a handbook for preceptors. Baillière Tindall, Edinburgh.
Stuart C 2004 Assessment, supervision and support in clinical practice: a guide for nurses, midwives and other health professionals. Churchill Livingstone, Edinburgh.

The Royal College of Nursing's *Clinical placement toolkit* is also a very good resource for mentors.

Appendix 1 NURSING AND MIDWIFERY COUNCIL QA FACTSHEET O/2003

NMC requirements for mentors and mentorship

Synopsis

1. This factsheet sets out the NMC standard for mentors and mentorship. It provides advice and guidance on the development of preparation programmes and gives information on how the NMC will quality assure its mentor standard. Finally, it identifies current action to develop mentor standards in response to changes in regulation and education provision.

2. The NMC has commenced a review of the teacher standards, including those for mentors and mentorship. It is anticipated that a draft standard will be published for wider consultation early in 2004.

Background

3. Whilst the UKCC set a standard for mentors, arrangements for the approval and monitoring of preparation programmes was for the previous National Boards to determine. Mentor qualifications are not, and never have been, recorded on the register. Whereas some National Boards previously granted awards for these programmes, the NMC would now expect Higher Education Institutions (HEIs) to have their own register of approved mentors.

4. On 1 April 2002, when the NMC formally came into being, the Council adopted all extant UKCC and National Board regulations and standards. Previously a tripartite letter had been issued for England by the DH/UKCC/ENB identifying that those post-registration programmes that did not lead to registration or a recordable qualification would become the business of Higher Education Institutions in partnership with service providers. This identified that extant standards would continue to inform such programmes until replaced by NMC standards.

The status of mentor standards

5. The current standard for mentors and mentorship is included within the NMC publication *Standard for the preparation of teachers of nursing and midwifery* (NMC 2002) and is identified as an advisory standard. It is presented in the form of outcomes to be met.

6. In March 2003, Council agreed that the status of mentorship standards should change from advisory to required. A letter

informed HEIs of this change and provided advice (QA9 July 2003).

Requirements of the current mentor standards

7. Nurses and midwives who take on the role of mentor must have current registration with the NMC. This includes second level registered nurses. They will have completed at least twelve months full time post-qualifying experience (or equivalent part-time). They should receive support from qualified nurse and midwife teachers and experienced practitioners in carrying out their mentor role.

NMC guidance for preparing mentors

8. The NMC advises a flexible approach toward preparation of mentors that involves learning in both practice and academic environments in order to meet the required outcomes. Programme providers, HEIs and their service partners, should agree an approach that is designed to meet both local needs and NMC requirements.

9. The NMC does not require a specific academic level for mentorship preparation. Council requires that pre-registration programmes must be a minimum of Diploma of Higher Education and that Specialist Practice Qualifications be at no less than degree level. Therefore the expectation would be that mentorship programmes would be set at an appropriate academic level.

10. It would be a matter for HEIs and their service partners to justify the mode and level of mentor preparation at approval events for programmes leading to registration or recordable qualifications.

11. Programme providers should consider how accreditation of prior (experiential) learning (AP(E)L) might be used to bring all mentors to an equitable level of preparation in meeting the NMC requirements. This would allow those who have undertaken short preparation programmes, alternative programmes such as for assessing NVQ/SVQ, or developed their competence through experience to reach a comparable standard to those undertaking a contemporary preparation programme.

Guidance for updating mentors

12. Programme providers should develop a process for updating mentors on a regular basis. The NMC requires regular updating of mentors.

Quality assurance arrangements

13. The effect of the change in status of the mentor standard enables NMC Visitors in England, and agents in Northern Ireland, Scotland and Wales, to require evidence that NMC mentorship outcomes have been met by those undertaking this role. A document mapping the local preparation programme against NMC outcomes for mentorship would be helpful in clarifying this for the Visitor/Agent.

14. During annual monitoring the NMC Visitor/Agent would seek evidence that there were sufficient numbers of appropriately prepared mentors to support students studying for registration or recordable qualifications. They would also seek evidence that there had been relevant and regular opportunities for mentors to update their knowledge and skills in order to maintain and develop their competence.

September 2003

Appendix 2 LEARNING CONTRACT

In this example, the student has had just over 2 weeks to prepare to give a presentation on an aspect of infection control. The student will be evaluated based on her knowledge and understanding of key elements of infection control. To prepare for this, the student and mentor make a plan to help the student identify and research in preparation for the seminar. This learning contract helps the student to reach the learning outcome. Many portfolios and documents sent out by the university will have learning outcomes broken into steps, but learning contracts are very good for learning complex skills or concepts.

Learning contract

Student name: Rahma Ahmed   Date: 10 May 2007

Learning outcome: The student will demonstrate understanding of infection control. To meet this outcome, the student will:

- Identify resources and policy that inform and guide the nurse.
- Identify common microorganisms, their signs and symptoms, diseases they cause, and discuss their transmission.
- Discuss the rationale for and practice of infection control techniques, considering various methods of transmission.
- Give a brief presentation on infection control at a staff meeting on 27 May 2007.

Table 7.1

Intervention	Time frame	Completed
Visit library and identify relevant journals and books, and electronic resources	11 May	Identified three journals, two books and two websites
Attend Infection Control Study day	13 May	Attended study day and received Trust literature and policy
Discussion with mentor and with Infection Control Nurse	13 May	Mentor suggested looking at MRSA, E. coli, TB and Pseudomonas. Infection control nurse said many nurses don't really understand air-borne transmission
Make a list of common microorganisms that cause clinical infections, outline the signs/symptoms/transmission of each	13–17 May	Used the journal articles and books to make outline. Written down what they look like, how they are diagnosed and what they do. Found good article on TB and airborne transmission. Would make a good presentation
Outline methods of transmission, and how transmission can be prevented	17–19 May	Have looked at transmission and broken transmission into categories: air-borne, blood-borne and direct contact. Will review list with mentor. **Good job! I.S. 18 May**
Identify ways infection control is maintained in the clinical environment	10–27 May	Have had meeting with Infection Control Nurse again and trudged through all the infection control policies, applying them to what I found out about transmission
Infection control presentation at staff meeting	27 May	Presentation done on air-borne infection. Made a chart for ward on different organisms. **Well done Rahma! I.S.**
Demonstrate appropriate professional hygiene	11–27 May	Have been washing hands, using hand gel, aprons, etc. and maintaining general cleanliness. **Agreed I.S.**

Evaluation: Rahma has been diligent and thorough, did an excellent and relevant presentation, and has been consistently demonstrating her knowledge in her practice. Well done!

Imana Sessorand, Mentor
27 May 2007

8 Pitfalls in practice

- Burnout and stress
- Bullying and harassment
- Dealing with difficult people
- Whistleblowing and preventing fraud
- Health and safety concerns
- Debt and financial problems
- 'The smell of burning martyr'
- Summary

This chapter discusses some of the more difficult parts of nursing – dealing with difficult situations and difficult people. Believe it or not, the most important skill you will develop when growing into an experienced nurse is how to cope with difficult stress and with difficult people.

Taking care of your patients means taking care of yourself: in this chapter you will find information about avoiding some of those problems that can make you miserable at work.

BURNOUT AND STRESS

'Stress' really isn't a very good word to use – it has such a negative connotation! In reality, stress is something we live with every day. It helps us make good decisions, it keeps our minds sharp. A life without stress would be boring and dull.

The problem with 'stress' isn't the stress itself – it's the way we cope (or don't cope) with it. When we use up all of our coping mechanisms (the good ones and the bad ones) and have nothing left, then we enter burnout. Like ashes in the fireplace, being burned out means having everything that's good, all the energy, all the potential, destroyed.

When we are burned out, we don't make very good partners, friends or parents; we don't make very good nurses either. That's the real tragedy of trying too hard and doing too much – the more you drive yourself to do the impossible, the more impossible it becomes and eventually all the people you were working so hard for are too much effort to keep up relationships with. If you burn out, the compassion, kindness and knowledge that give your nursing its special touch will disappear like smoke up a chimney.

So how can we prevent getting burned out by too much stress?

First thing is that you must make a commitment to being healthy, inside and out. You start to feel stressed, and cope with it much less effectively, if you aren't well. You have to take care of yourself if you are going to have the energy to take care of others.

Time for a story . . .

Midori was a Japanese nurse studying for her registration exams in America. One day, during a hectic week of preparation for the difficult exams, her room-mate Alice found her outside sitting in the sun. Her placid face made it look as if she hadn't a care in the world.

Alice went outside in a huff. 'You have so much to do! Why are you wasting all this time, you haven't got it to waste!'

Midori calmly took off her sunglasses and smiled. 'I am not wasting time, I am recharging my energy. I am solar powered!' As she put her sunglasses back on, Alice marched back inside the building and, an hour later when Midori came back into the room, she was frantic and in an absolute state. Midori quietly gathered her books and sat on her bed, reading her material.

The next day, the two girls were discussing the exam for which they had been preparing. Midori said she was confident that she had done well but Alice was very disappointed in her performance. She said 'All the time I put in studying and I can't remember anything. You spent half the time, and you did well.'

Midori replied 'You studied in a thunderstorm, your mind full of lightning and the wind blowing your thoughts all over. I studied in a warm summer breeze, and planted my thoughts neatly in orderly rows. When I went to look for my thoughts, they were there waiting. You had to study **and** fight the storm – I only had to study.'

Midori had a secret – she knew that if she allowed herself some time, she would be able to think more clearly and so would use her time more efficiently. The same is true of qualified nurses – if you allow yourself to get frustrated then you will have two problems: whatever it is you have to deal with and the problems you make for yourself by the way you are dealing with it.

If you are low on sleep, powered by junk food and have been working too many hours, then you will not have the reserve you need to step back and relax. You have to recognise that you are a nurse – not a superhero – and that you can't take care of anyone else if you aren't physically taking care of yourself.

Physical well-being isn't just about joining a gym or being on a diet – it can be going for walks, doing garden work, eating fruit and vegetables, cutting down on alcohol, getting enough sleep – all of these things can help you.

Next, you have to take care of yourself emotionally. Nursing is a demanding job and we are constantly exposed to the fears, pain and suffering of other people. We try so hard to be everything other people need us to be and, when we simply can't do it all, we start to feel guilty and frustrated.

If we make mistakes, or things don't go well, we turn inward and blame ourselves. We want to fix things – and it's hard to accept, as a professional problem-fixer, that there are some things that just must stay broken.

As nurses, we find it difficult to convince our hearts to accept that sometimes people die, that sometimes people seem to have been dealt very unfair hands in life, and that as nurses sometimes we can only stand by as nature takes its course. We know with our minds that it's part of the work we do, but our hearts get hurt. This shakes our confidence and makes it even more difficult.

Then, because we think that it's weakness to be upset, we bottle it up and try to hide it. The truth is that talking about how you feel can make it easier to cope. Sometimes you need to have a good cry, or a good moan, and get it out of your system.

Finally, you need to take care of yourself socially. You can't survive if you are working so much that you don't spend time with family and friends; you must spend time with people you love and who love you. You have to keep interests and hobbies, and you have to spend time away from nursing. Working bank holiday shifts should not be your hobby!

Research shows that the best way to beat stress and burnout is to have a healthy social life – friends and family are the medicine that keeps us well.

One of the greatest skills you develop as a nurse is key to preventing burnout and stress: communication. You don't have to go into gory details, or divulge confidential details, but talking to people about your work and how you feel can help you. Have a laugh with other nurses, get involved in causes that interest you – remember that no matter how tough things get, you are never alone as a nurse. There are millions of us out here all over the world and all of us, at one time or another, go through a difficult patch.

Reaching out

Another way to beat stress is to reach out to others:

● Does your organisation have an activities department? A day centre? A creche? Could you help out, donate something, donate time?
● Does your organisation have links with organisations like the Royal National Institute for the Blind, Age Concern, the Multiple Sclerosis Society? Could you spare a couple of hours and volunteer?

As a nurse, you have many different types of skill: communication and helping are two of the biggies. Are you willing to help others? Can you reach out a little further? Volunteering makes you feel good and is an excellent way to beat stress. It's also a fun way to meet people, to meet your post-registration education and practice (PREP) obligations and to expand your network and professional knowledge. Give it a try.

Where I work, we have an active crafts and activities department. The facilitator is a miracle-worker. She gives people hope, company, distraction from pain and all kinds of problems and, in the process, gets people to knit blankets for the dog and cat shelters, make cards to sell to raise more money for crafts and helps people find new talents and skills. She is wonderful and I always bring things in for her to use. Are there skills you could share to make the world better for those for whom you care?

Perhaps you are a specialist nurse? Could you provide your skill in another country as part of a medical mission?

I know you are busy, but would an hour or two really break the bank? Try volunteering to beat your stress and make the world brighter.

What can you do if it starts getting more than you can bear?

Get help – no one is going to think you weak, just sensible for knowing when you need help:

● go to your GP
● go to your occupational health department
● the NMC has an advice line
● both Unison and the RCN have free counselling available for members
● take a Tai-Chi, meditation or relaxation class
● plan some time off with family and friends.

These are just a few possible ideas . . . but don't just hide waiting for things to get better. Hiding and avoiding the way you are feeling may work in the short term, but it makes things much worse – and much more difficult – in the long run.

What are the symptoms of stress overload?

- Loss of appetite.
- Food cravings when under pressure.
- Frequent tummy upsets.
- Constipation or diarrhoea.
- Problems sleeping (too much or too little).
- Feeling worried or anxious but not knowing why.
- Being snappy or short with people.
- Withdrawing from things you used to enjoy.
- Just not caring any more.

Burnout costs the NHS millions of pounds in sick days and lost productivity, and it costs nurses and other healthcare professionals much more on personal levels. Be the kind of nurse your patient needs you to be – be *healthy*.

You became a nurse to take care of people who need you – remember: you need you too!

One kind of problem that causes a considerable amount of stress in the workplace is bullying and harassment.

BULLYING AND HARASSMENT

Theresa is a nurse on a busy ward. She doesn't get on very well with her manager and this is making her miserable. She goes to her manager and tells her that she would like their working relationship to be better. The manager tells her that she doesn't see it as a problem and therefore doesn't see that anything can be done. She suggests Theresa gets counselling for her 'paranoia'.

After this meeting, Theresa finds herself getting all the tough assignments and shifts. She is working more weekends and bank holidays than anyone else, and she was already feeling very burned out because she was working night shifts so often.

Theresa feels as though she can't do anything right: although the manager isn't specifically saying anything bad, her actions are making Theresa feel unfairly treated. When she raises her concerns again, her manager says that, as Theresa is the most senior nurse, she is needed at all these times because the manager relies on her so heavily.

The manager doesn't think anything is wrong but Theresa is ready to quit: is she being bullied? Theresa thinks so.

The key to bullying is that it's in the eye of the beholder; it's how the victim feels that matters. Some people won't feel bullied in a situation in which someone else will. A manager has to be sensitive to the way in which different people react to their guidance and management.

Do you think Theresa was being bullied?

Bullying

Let's look at what bullying is: bullying is when inadequate and insecure people try to make themselves feel better by making other people look or feel inadequate. This is done through criticism, lies, manipulation and humiliation.

Bullying is social and emotional violence: it is aggressive, antisocial behaviour that is protected by the bully spinning an intricate shield of denial, victimhood, manipulation and charm. It can escalate into physical violence, although, more often, the bully relies on threats and intimidation. Bullying can be direct but is most commonly a subterfuge that undermines and destroys people by whom the bully is threatened.

How do these people threaten the bully? By being competent, caring, successful people: there is nothing a bully likes less than to see someone doing or feeling better than he or she is.

What kind of people are the victims of bullies? You might think it's the weak, spineless person but in reality it's exactly the opposite. Someone who is weak isn't a threat – it's the strong person that scares a bully and so it's the strong person that the bully tries to knock down.

> Both seeking something precious, a thief empties the purse and a bully the soul . . .

If people who are bullied are strong people, what kind of people are bullies? Bullies are people who don't know how to cope with the world fairly, on even terms. Bullies are people who use power and aggression to get their way because they really don't think they have anything else to use. You can't reason with bullies and you can't get them to stop by showing them what they are doing to you – they don't care.

People who have to bully other people are weak, selfish and insecure, and have very poor self-esteem. Otherwise, they wouldn't need to make other people feel bad. Bullies are angry and bitter and want other people to feel as badly as they do.

Bullies are masters of deception and know how to turn on the charm when it will give credibility to their behaviour. They can be the most charismatic person imaginable – if others find it hard to believe that someone so charming could be a bully then they have longer to victimise others.

Bullies have many different ways of behaving, but the best way to know you are being bullied is:

- Do you *feel* bullied? Are you finding that you are losing confidence and self-esteem and that you are feeling anxious and worried?

That's the real test of bullying: if you feel like you are being bullied, are losing confidence and self-esteem, and are having anxiety, then you *are* being bullied.

What can you do?

- Realise that this is not your fault, there is nothing you have done to deserve it and it is not fair.
- Realise that there is nothing wrong with you.
- Realise that the bully is a malicious and inadequate person who can only hurt you if you let him or her.
- Tell the bully that you are no longer willing to accept his or her behaviour. If the person has power (such as a manager), then ask someone from your union or another friend to support you.
- Document what the person does and pursue a complaint if necessary.

The most powerful thing to say to a bully is 'I will not accept you treating me this way any longer', if you really mean it.

Being bullied is one of the most frightening things in the world, but as soon as you stand up to the bully you will feel that lost confidence and self-esteem return.

Bullies can only thrive when someone is willing to be a victim.

It is possible that someone – say a new manager, or someone from a different culture – might feel that they are being assertive or strong by behaving as they do, but you are feeling bullied by their behaviour. That's why it's important that you speak up as soon as possible: if it's a genuine misunderstanding, it will be easier to sort out if you speak up sooner rather than later. If it is bullying, the sooner it stops, the better.

Harassment

Harassment and bullying are really very similar: bullying can often be a kind of harassment, and harassment can be bullying. It doesn't matter what you call it, as long as you recognise when you are not being treated fairly and with respect.

Harassment is when something happens and it isn't welcome. It is an event or series of events that cause you to feel upset, belittled or threatened.

Harassment affects the dignity and personhood of the individual being harassed, and can be focused on any aspect of that person:

- age
- gender
- race
- personal characteristics (tall, fat, thin, bald, etc.)
- disability
- national origin
- religion or belief.

It can be a one-off event or a series of events. It can be done face to face, over the phone, anonymously, even in e-mails. Did you know that sending a sexually related joke through e-mail could be construed as harassment if someone reads it and is offended?

Sometimes it is obvious that a person is being targeted:

- inappropriate touching or sexual conduct
- inappropriate comments
- malicious rumours or gossip
- insults.

Sometimes it is less obvious:

- being overly critical
- treating people unfairly
- excluding someone
- being openly critical
- picking on someone
- theft
- vandalism
- 'jokes' that demean or belittle a particular group
- rude cartoons or pictures.

Sometimes, it can be made to look 'supportive' or like assertive management:

- being very critical of work performance even when that perfor-mance is competent
- threatening job security or advancement
- choosing one person who is favoured over another
- scheduling someone unfairly.

As in bullying, the person being harassed might be afraid that others will think he or she is weak, so keeps a stiff upper lip and tries to live through it. If the person harassing is more powerful or has more authority it can be very difficult to speak up – but speaking up is what you need to do.

If you feel like you are being belittled because of who you are, then you need to speak up.

Discrimination and harassment are not things that only happen from one group to another – it's not a racial thing and it's not a male/female thing – it's about one person or group of people making others feel less worthy because of their differences, whatever those differences might be.

CHECK YOURSELF: WHICH OF THESE THINGS WOULD BE HARASSMENT?

- Giving someone three weekends in a row in the off duty so your friend can have an extra weekend off.
- Calling someone a 'damn Yankee'.
- Telling sexually explicit jokes.
- Telling a joke like 'An Englishman, an Irishman and a Scotsman walk into a bar . . .' (just so you know, the rest of that story is 'They each order a pint and then catch the bus home. The joke is that the bus is on time).
- Patting a colleague's bottom.
- Asking an Asian colleague if she had an arranged marriage.
- Constantly asking a colleague for a date even when that colleague has said a clear 'No'.

All of these things could be harassment:
   Harassment is:

- unwelcome
- belittling to the personal dignity of a person
- based on a personal characteristic or feature
- one event or a series of events.

Although it can be scary, you have to speak up: harassment will get worse before it gets better if allowed to continue. Your employer should have guidelines on addressing bullying and harassment: You have a right to work in an environment free from risk and hazard – that means you have a right to work free from bullying and harassment.

   The following contacts can help you:

- **Commission for Racial Equality:** tackles racial discrimination and promotes racial equality. Tel 020 7939 0000, website: http://www. cre.gov.uk

- **Disability Rights Commission:** provides information and advice to disabled people and employers about their rights and duties. Tel 08457 622 633, website: http://www.drc.org.uk
- **Equal Opportunities Commission:** works to eliminate sex discrimination. Tel 08456 015 901, website: http://www.eoc.org.uk

You can also contact your union and your human resources department.

DEALING WITH DIFFICULT PEOPLE

Some skills will always work with difficult people. The real thing is to manage your expectations of the difficult person!

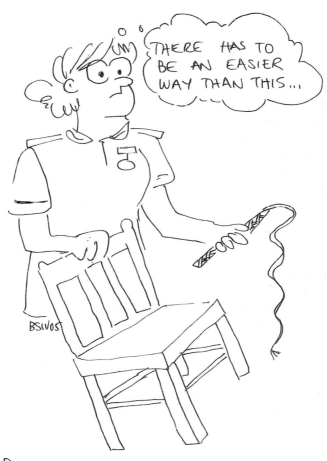

DEALING WITH DIFFICULT PEOPLE IS EASIER THAN IT MAY SEEM.

There is an old Polish saying: 'Only a fool expects a horse to bark.' This is a reminder that once you know how someone will react, it's silly to expect them to behave differently. What you need to do is know how to divert, deflect and settle the behaviours the person uses to be so difficult.

Let's look first how to deal with people who are actively, in-your-face difficult:

> A member of a patient's family has come to speak with you. She is angry – really angry – and is screaming at you. She will not calm down and will not listen . . . and you need to think fast.

What do you do?

- Speak in a quiet, measured tone of voice: do not match the other person's tempo, volume or speed.
- Smile and use open body language.
- Agree with the person whenever possible: there is nothing more disarming to an angry person than for someone to say 'Yes, that's right, I agree.'
- If you were in the wrong (even just a little bit), acknowledge this and say you are sorry: 'Yes, I agree, we should have called you. You are right; I am sorry and I was wrong not to call you.' It is commonly believed that saying sorry means you are accepting liability for the mistake. This is wrong; it does not.
- Write down what the person is saying. Tell her: 'I want to make sure I get this right because it's obviously important to you'. Use empathetic feedback (more on this later) to show you understand.
- Sit down. Get the other person to sit down. Be civil and patient. Offer a cup of tea.
- Give your name and call them Mr or Mrs unless they ask you to call them by the first name.

You also might want to make sure that someone calls security, the Matron or someone else in case the matter escalates.

Some things never to do are:

- Never go head-to-head: it's foolhardy and unprofessional.
- Never try to drown-out the other person.
- Never make it worse by accusing the other person of making things worse.
- Never get yourself in a situation where the angry person is between you and the way out.

- Never try to handle a person like this all alone: make sure someone knows you need help.

Some people are difficult in a way that is not in your face but behind your back. For example:

Jojesh is a computer programmer in the finance directorate. He is the most skilled of a group of programmers. He knows that he is more skilled and knowledgeable than most, so he feels a great deal of job security.

He doesn't make friends with the people at work. He comes in late and will leave mid-sentence when the clock strikes 5. He takes extended lunch breaks, more sick days than anyone else and often ignores requests for help. He will throw things in the bin right in front of you if he doesn't want to do them.

Alison works with Jojesh and she is fed up with being treated badly. She goes to her manager and complains. Jojesh is told that he should be nicer and friendlier but he resents this. He starts to complain about how women whine when they are 'unfulfilled'. Alison is furious! She comes to you for help.

What do you say?

- Think about a horse barking: what can you expect from Jojesh?
- Is there really anything Alison can do herself?
- Is there anything anyone else can do, other than the manager?

Alison should keep a log, looking at every interaction she has with Jojesh. She should reflect on every occurrence, always making abso-lutely certain that she isn't even a tiny part of the problem. She can confront Jojesh, but it's unlikely to work because he isn't very respectful.

She should not get into a gossip war or start talking about him behind his back. His actions speak loudly without her help. If she starts badmouthing him then he has an excuse for the way he acts.

So, let's see what we know about dealing with difficult people now:

- Reflect on your interactions with them.
- Keep a log.
- Don't make yourself look bad by engaging in bad behaviours your-self, like gossiping or backstabbing.
- Recognise when you are powerless over someone else's behaviour.

- Always behave in a discreet, polite and respectable way so no one has grounds to blame their behaviour on you.

Empathetic listening and feedback

This is useful when dealing with someone who is complaining and very angry. Listen to what they say. Here is a typical 'rant' you might hear:

> I was told to be here to pick up my wife at 2 p.m. but she's not ready. And it costs £1 an hour to park in the car park. This is all about getting money, isn't it! Do you get commission? Is that why you make me wait? What have you been doing all day – why can't you get my wife ready? Are you hiding something? Is she unwell? If you have let her catch some kind of superbug I'll sue. The Sister yesterday said . . .

Look at what the person is really saying:

- Someone in a uniform just like yours made a promise and you didn't keep it.
- I have needs and you are not meeting them.
- The fact you didn't keep your promise is costing me time and money.

That's empathetic listening. It means listening to the feelings and thoughts, not just the words. It means putting yourself in the other person's shoes and allowing yourself to see how they see the situation.

Now for the feedback part: 'Sir, you're right. She should have been ready. I could tell you how busy we are, but that doesn't change the fact that your wife isn't ready. I'm sorry'.

People yell only when they think no-one is listening. You will take away the need to yell if you prove you are listening.

The next step is helping to solve whatever problems you recognise that the person you are dealing with feels you have caused. In this case it is:

- wife not ready
- car park charge.

Perhaps his wife is waiting for records to be signed off, which is totally beyond your control. Be honest, but don't let it sound like an excuse: 'Sir, your wife needs a document signed by the consultant and he is late for rounds; that is the reason for the delay.'

Now, apply some creative problem solving and critical thinking: is there any way around this? Can the man and his wife come back for whatever it is that needs to be signed? Can it be posted? Can you get a verbal approval instead of the signature? Can you get the car parking fees waived?

Imagine – will the man still be yelling if he hears: 'Sir, you are right . . . she should have been ready. I can explain why if you want to hear but the end result is that it's not fair you have been left here waiting. The form needs to be signed before we can discharge your wife, but if you would like to go for a cup of tea, both of you, in the canteen, one of the nurses will come down and tell you as soon as the notes are signed and then you can leave. And I will call security and ask if they can let you out of the car park without paying a charge as you are right, it's not fair. Is there anything else I can do to make it up to you both? Your wife is so lovely and it has been so wonderful to care for her, I hate for her to have such a bad last day with us . . .'

Just remember to follow through on anything you promise. And see what I snuck in at the end? That's the offer of a win–win, another significant tool in dealing with difficult people.

Win–win?

Yes. It's the place where both people get benefit. What the nurse was offering when she said 'Your wife is so lovely and it has been so wonderful to care for her, I hate for her to have such a bad last day with us . . .' was: Look, we know we messed up but you haven't been easy either. Let's both be good so your wife doesn't get upset, as she is innocent in all this and this will upset her needlessly.

A win–win isn't always possible but, if it is, it is helpful to use. Try to find a place where both people can feel good about the outcome. Try to make a peaceful resolution where there is no blame or shame. In this case, it also gives the man a chance to calm down and save face. No-one likes to feel put down or ashamed of their behaviour. The truth is that you know he's a jerk, he knows he's a jerk and neither of you needs to rub it in.

Later, he might even come to you and say 'You know, I was a bit hot-headed earlier . . .' and the best type of reaction is to say something like 'Thank you, but I understand, you love your wife, and you have been so worried and stressed by all of this . . . I'm glad I could help'.

There is never a win in saying something that takes away the chance for the person to save face. How would it sound for the nurse to say: 'Hot headed? A total jerk, more like. You're lucky I didn't call Security to bounce you out of here . . .'. Unprofessional and uncaring, that's how. It doesn't matter if the whole world doesn't know how unfairly you were treated. What's important is your patient. Being kind and forgiving to this patient's husband helps your patient; isn't that what you would want if the roles were reversed?

Remember: Giving people a chance to win, and to save face, will improve their odds of gong with what you suggest.

OK, so we have looked at screaming people and people who are aggressive in a passive sort of way, let's look at a few others.

Say it all – do nothing

Some people promise the world but deliver nothing. These people get onto committees, eat the food, drink the coffee, sign up for everything and never deliver. At the deadline, there is always an excuse or reason and nothing gets done.

- If you know people like this, resist the temptation to accept their help, even to the point of saying, privately 'Thanks for the offer of help Theresa, but last time you said you would help you didn't, and I had a lot of work to do at the last minute as a result'.
- If you must accept their help, have someone else work with them.
- Check up and ask for frequent progress reports, and ask for proof of work during the process.

If you are on a ward and a person like this is a healthcare assistant, you have a real problem: you need things to be done in short order and you don't have time to play games. You might want to work with this person directly so you can give him or her explicit directions ('You go and wash Mrs Bradley and then come back to me, in no more than 10 minutes') and notice when they are busy doing nothing ('Put that magazine down and come help me please').

A variant of this type of person is the 'fag-break ghost'. This is the person who takes a lot of breaks, and they are all too long. People like this really erode morale because everyone does their work for them. They also make other people late for *their* breaks. The only way to deal with someone like this is to say 'You have your break at 10 a.m. and at 1.15 in the afternoon. Your breaks are 10 minutes. You must be back here at 10.10 a.m. and at 1.25 p.m.' State your expectations clearly. If the person still doesn't listen, set your limit: 'If you are late from your next break, I will write this up. It's a shame because you work so hard but the excessiveness of your breaks is out of control, and I need you to work hard because we are busy and you are capable of so much . . .'

- Be specific in your expectations.
- Set limits if you feel taken advantage of, and follow through when you say you will.

- Don't let anyone else talk you into 'one more chance' when you know that the person has had his or her last chance over and over again.
- In general, it's always useful to phrase things in a 'critical sandwich': take a good thing, then the problem, then a good thing – it makes the problem easier to swallow. Can you find the sandwich in the paragraph above?

The intimidator

Some people use threats and intimidation to get their way; the threats can be direct or indirect. Here is an example of an indirect intimidator:

Carla is a manager of a day hospital. She is a very intimidating person but is careful to always say everything with a smile and use all the right words. Under the words, the message is very clear: my way or the highway.

One day, she finds an incomplete expense report on a secretary's desk. She knows it is for items paid for out of ward funds, and that those funds are adequate to pay for this expense. She also knows that the secretary had permission to buy the items, but she has had a bad day and wants to kick the dog. She calls the ward manager who will deal with the request and says 'Hello, how are you? How was your holiday? You know, budgets are very tight and I don't see how we can pay these . . . it's a shame you didn't talk to me about them. I'll get rid of them for you, and please come see me in the future . . .

What do you do?

- Keep a log.
- Reflect on how this person makes you feel.
- Get help in dealing with the way this person makes you feel.
- Stand up for yourself: 'Carla, that expense report is incomplete and it's perfectly fine; those items have already been approved. Do not get rid of it, please put it back where it belonged. Thank you'.
- Don't show that you have been upset, shaken or stirred: the more this kind of person knows that what they do works, the more they do it. Smile, laugh, try 'Oh, you joker! You had me for a minute there! Ha ha! You know that is already approved to come out of ward funds, you really had me going! That was really funny, thanks for the laugh Carla!'.

The gossip

Gossips find out and share, or make up and share, details about other people. They say things like 'You know what I heard?' or 'Guess what!' or 'Wait until you hear!'. These people make others feel on edge because they don't usually share things like 'Beth wrote another book, aren't we proud of her?'; they say things like 'Oh heavens, did you see what Lynne was wearing into work? Can you believe it? Charity shop special Ha ha ha.'

These people are hurtful and they drag other people in. Be absolutely sure that at the first opportunity they will use the fact that you listened to get them out of trouble. 'Lynn, I was speaking to Beth, and I don't mean to be hurtful but she was making some nasty remarks about you . . .'

Your only defence against gossips is not to engage in gossip. Ever. And to let gossips know that it is not welcome.

The mouse

The mouse is the last person in the world anyone would want to speak up to. They are quiet, shy, almost painfully vague and incapable. They hardly ever speak up and even a gentle word of encouragement brings them to shed tears as they run away.

These people are clever: they know that you are a nice person and you don't want to hurt them; they run away knowing most people are uncomfortable chasing them, and most people don't want to get into 'painful' conversations.

Some techniques that work with mice are:

- 'OK, I see you are upset. Come back in 10 minutes so we can finish our talk.'
- Then, go find the person in 10 minutes.

These people might need the ward or team manager to bring them into accountability but the most important thing for you to remember is that you are not to be ignored, or made to look evil, by someone who is trying to avoid responsibility. Some people are not acting like mice – they are really shy. You can tell the difference: are they always shy or only when someone has to say something difficult to them?

In summary

You will encounter many difficult people; some of whom will be more difficult than others. Some will be loud and difficult, some quiet and difficult. Some will be manipulative, some will be bullies, some will be gossips. The information I have already given you will help, so let's go over the most important tips overall:

- Treat everyone with respect, dignity and fairness. Praise in public and criticise in private.
- Look for and offer win–wins and opportunities to save face.
- Keep your tone, volume, body language and posture neutral: be calm and open.
- Don't expect anyone to behave differently than they have before. Only a fool expects a horse to bark!
- Say sorry if it helps the other person hear and listen.
- Agree with the other person if he or she is right.
- Show you are interested in people by writing down what they say.
- Use empathetic listening and feedback.
- Solve whatever problems you can, this can help to calm complainers.
- Set limits when necessary to settle-down people who take advantage or whose behaviour is disruptive.
- Get help if you might be unsafe or unable to manage alone.
- Think: which is more important: being right or living peacefully?, and act accordingly.
- Treat people and behave as you wish to be treated and have people behave around you.
- People who are difficult to deal with need compassion, caring and limits.
- By not being a person who is difficult yourself, you make it easier for everyone else as they have one less difficult person to deal with.

WHISTLEBLOWING AND PREVENTING FRAUD

All NHS Trusts have a policy on whistleblowing.

Whistleblowing is when a person stands up and lets others know that a dangerous, illegal or unfair practice is going on. The person 'blowing the whistle' is like the match referee holding up a red card and saying 'That's not on, and you can't do that here'.

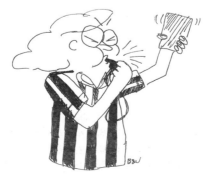

There are some common areas that people raise:

- health and safety
- fraud
- abuse
- care issues
- discrimination and harassment
- unfair or illegal practices.

Whistleblowing is more than just raising a complaint. People who complain have encountered the problem themselves – a customer, a patient, an innocent bystander. Someone who whistleblows is usually coming from within an organisation and is concerned that something the organisation, or someone within the organisation, is doing is somehow wrong.

SOME WHISTLEBLOWING: CASES FROM THE MEDIA

- A cleaner at a chemical company alerted the police when he realised that toxic chemicals were being poured into the drains.
- A nurse alerted hospital administration when she realised that another member of staff was very aggressive with vulnerable clients.
- A member of staff in a large company alerted police about postal fraud – the company was shipping things in a way to avoid VAT.

Being a whistleblower means taking a stand to make sure that the right things happen. It is a way of protecting the public.

As a nurse, you have an obligation under the NMC *Code of professional conduct* to speak up if you realise that something is not right. You have an obligation to protect the public. In fact, there is even a law to help whistleblowers: the Public Interest Disclosure Act 1998 (PIDA). The PIDA protects employees who raise concerns about their organisation's actions or practices.

Speaking up

A common area in which you might need to speak up is in clinical practice. What do you do when you see improper clinic activity? Lack of hand-washing? Failure to check identification before giving medication? It's up to you, either you go ahead and say something yourself or you talk to a senior staff member. The place you work can only give care as well as the weakest member of staff. Protecting patients and staff means speaking up. It's not as dramatic as whistleblowing but it's just as important.

Preventing fraud: an important part of whistleblowing

You might know that something is wrong in your area, your ward, your hospital or your Trust, but what about the NHS as a whole? What kinds of things do you think harm the NHS:

- Taking an occasional ream of photocopy paper home with you.
- Faking documentation to cover work you didn't do.
- Claiming for mileage you didn't use.
- Claiming for expenses you didn't incur.
- Using a friend's company to provide a business service and artificially elevating costs.
- Taking scissors or a book from the ward.

All of these things are bad; they all cost the NHS money and prevent resources being available when they are needed.

You can contact the NHS Fraud line or a manager in your organisation if you are concerned about fraud.

In summary

Have you ever parked in disabled parking 'just for a minute' – what about the person who really needed that space? Ever wear a uniform that should have been laundered? Worse yet, worn it out in public, in the market or in a pub? Ever taken someone else's lunch out of the ward fridge? These things not only hurt people, they could harm patients and they destroy trust. You have to be above question as someone who would do the respectable, legal and responsible thing.

Finally, about whistleblowing in general:

- Speaking up and saying 'I don't think that is right' promotes respect in general. Remember, the *Code of professional conduct* says that, as nurses, we must be the kind of person others look up to and respect because we are trustworthy.
- Speaking up and blowing the whistle might mean challenging staff, visitors and sometimes – with support – even patients. It might mean challenging the entire organisation and risking your job. Only you can decide how far to go.

If you suspect that you need to 'blow the whistle', you should contact a union steward, someone in the human resources department or even someone at the NMC on the advice line.

If it's an issue of fraud, contact the NHS Fraud and corruption helpline on 08702 400 100.

HEALTH AND SAFETY CONCERNS

As a nurse, you might find there are times when you are asked to do things in ways you know they shouldn't be done. However, you:

- should always use the correct personal protection equipment
- should use manual handling aids
- should not do any inappropriate lifting or moving
- should not carry sharps from their place of use to a bin.

However, we all know that – unfortunately – people take shortcuts with health and safety. Perhaps it is not their intention to behave in an unsafe manner but people in clinical practice say the following kinds of things too often:

- 'Don't bother with the hoist, we can just lift her'
- 'I left the sharps bin in my car/in the treatment room, so I will recap this needle'
- 'I don't need gloves – it's just a little bit of wee!'

There are two reasons you must take health and safety seriously:

1. **It's about protecting people:** yourself, patients, family/carers, the general public and colleagues.
2. **The law states you must comply with health and safety legislation** and the NMC *Code of professional conduct* implies you must comply with law. A failure to follow health and safety procedures could lead to disciplinary problems, lost wages and perhaps even the loss of your right to practise.

There are some other potential health and safety pitfalls you should look out for:

- **Hand-washing:** this works only if you do it properly. Failure to properly wash hands is one of the most significant factors in the transmission of disease. Be kind to your hands – dry them thoroughly and use a moisturiser.
- **Hand gel:** this is increasingly being used when hand-washing isn't convenient but, again, it only works if used properly. You should spread hand gel over your hands the same way you wash them – not just the palms but the entire hands, between fingers, the back of the hands, etc. Also, hand gel is potentially flammable; if you store it in the boot of your car, it could pose a risk.
- **Latex:** healthcare professionals are at risk for developing latex allergies. You must be aware of your risk and use the most appropriate glove. If you don't need to use latex, you should consider alternatives.

- **Uniforms:** your uniform is a piece of personal protective equipment. It is intended to be worn once and laundered, and not to be worn outside the clinical areas. It could put others – and yourself! – at risk if you wear your uniform outside your clinical area. If you are a community nurse, you should be aware that just because you wear your uniform 'out and about' doesn't mean you should wear it to do your grocery shopping on the way home!
- **Aggression and violence:** although there is a 'zero tolerance' policy for aggression against healthcare workers, this can be very difficult to enforce. Some patients, because of their medical condition, can become verbally or physically violent. You still need to take care of such patients but if one starts to become difficult to manage, you should get help from a more senior member of staff. If you are working in an environment where an assault or aggression is more likely (A&E, the community, mental health, learning disabilities, prison, etc.) then you should consider your personal safety. Do you have a personal alarm? Phone? Should you consider taking self-defence lessons?
- **Exposure to disease:** as a nurse, you will be exposed to all kinds of germs that other people only get by being ill. HIV, meningitis, MRSA, maybe even TB – all things you will come into contact with at work, and they are not the only ones! You need to be scrupulously careful with your personal hygiene if you are to protect yourself and your family, as well as the public in general, from catching even a small 'bug' like a cold.

Health and safety is everyone's worry, and you must take it seriously. Taking shortcuts might seem easier at the moment, but in the long run they can seriously cost you.

DEBT AND FINANCIAL PROBLEMS

As a student, you were skint. You became a nurse and suddenly your pay increased and, if you are like everyone else, you started to spend more money. Before too long, you might have credit card bills and loans, and your pay isn't stretching as far as you would like.

So, you start working more shifts, a few hours here, a day there . . . but before too long even that money is getting used up. So you work more, and more . . . and then there is nothing left of you because you are all burned up.

If you are newly qualifying, wait until your financial situation stabilises before spending all kinds of money on things you could only dream of as a student – holidays, a car, renovations to your home, clothes. Wait: the cost is higher than you realise – do you want to give up all your free time to work to pay for these things?

You can often get financial advice from your union, from your employer and from Citizen's Advice bureaux. Don't let your finances hold you prisoner. Work so you can have a life outside work!

Another financial worry is the pension. The NHS Pensions Agency can give you advice about what your annual pension will be if you work in the NHS. If you don't work in the NHS you should speak to your human resources department. Even if you are a young person – in fact *especially* if you are a young person – you have to make certain that your pension will be sufficient. It might seem like a good idea to put the minimum amount into your pension fund, but in 40 years you will be sorry.

Financial advisors are making some pretty grim predications about pensions and poverty in old age – make sure that you take care of the future you.

'THE SMELL OF BURNING MARTYR'

What's the worst smell you get in healthcare? No matter how badly a body fluid might smell, the smell of burning martyr is always worse. Of course, the martyr wouldn't be happy if it wasn't the worst!

The martyr is the person who does too much, and loves it. Complain, whine, carry on – but never let up. The martyr is worried about problems, but not quite enough to offer solutions.

The martyr sees the bad side of everyone and everything. An optimist sees a glass half full, the pessimist sees the glass half empty and the martyr sees that as soon as someone else finishes their drink, he or she has yet another glass to wash!

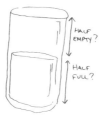

The martyr is a very destructive force in a clinical environment. This person can single-handedly prevent innovation and creative problem solving, adversely affect recruitment and retention, and make the general mood absolutely morbid.

> *Nurse A:* 'It's OK, I'll wash your cup.'
> *The martyr:* 'No, leave it, it's OK . . . (then after Nurse A leaves the
> cup) everyone else does . . .'

Or:

> *Nurse B:* 'Would you mind taking this late shift for me? I'll take
> one of yours . . .'
> *The martyr:* 'No problem, no need to switch, I'll just work it. I don't
> mind getting all the bad shifts.'
> *(Then later, to others):* 'Nurse B is having me work her late, and
> not even working one of mine . . . poor, poor me . . .'

'Poor me' is what martyrs are all about. They love being miserable, downtrodden and mistreated. They are death to good morale. If you have a martyr in your working environment, the best thing to do is avoid that person and not feed into his or her misery.

> *Nurse A:* 'It's OK, I'll wash your cup.'
> *The martyr:* 'No, leave it, it's OK . . . (then after Nurse A leaves the
> cup) everyone else does . . .'
> *Nurse A:* 'I think most people do clean up after themselves. Here,
> give me your cup, I'll wash it.'

And:

> *Nurse B:* 'Would you mind taking this late shift for me? I'll take
> one of yours . . .'
> *The martyr:* 'No problem, no need to switch, I'll just work it. I don't
> mind getting all the bad shifts.'
> *Nurse B:* Never mind then, I'll ask someone else.

The real tragedy of a martyr is that, usually, they were the person who once did do everything. They became so burned out that all they had left was complaining to keep them happy.

It is tempting to want to do too much – especially when you are new, you want to prove yourself and show you are a team player. But if you do too much, how are you going to get everything done well? At some point, you are going to be the one who is burned out, complaining and bringing everyone else down.

You need to be able to say 'No' when it is appropriate. Through reflection and clinical supervision you will learn where your limits and boundaries are, and what you need to do to keep yourself safe, sane and healthy.

Summary

- Nursing can be a stressful and demanding profession: you must be physically, emotionally and socially healthy if you are going to be the best nurse possible.
- Beating stress is possible – and sometimes, the way you beat stress can make the world a better place.
- No one has a right to make your life miserable and if you feel bullied or harassed the sooner you do something about it, the better.
- Bullying is in the eye of the beholder: if you feel bullied or harassed, you need to raise your concerns. It's not what someone says, it's what others *hear* that matters.
- You have professional, legal and moral obligations to speak up if you know something is wrong – although this is not always easy, it is something that simply has to happen. Because it can be difficult, there is support available to help you.
- You have professional and legal obligations to follow all health and safety guidance – shortcuts can cost you.
- 'Doing too much' can burn you out and turn you into a smouldering martyr who has nothing to do but complain and be miserable. Know your limits and get help when you need it.

9 Professional accountability and the NMC

- ● What is the NMC?
- ● Obligations and expectations of the professional nurse: the NMC *Code of professional conduct*
- ● Documentation and the guidelines for records and record keeping
- ● Medication administration and the guidelines for the administration of medications
- ● Summary
- ● Reference

WHAT IS THE NMC?

The Nursing and Midwifery Council (NMC) is an organisation that ensures nurses, midwives and specialist community public health nurses provide high standards of care to their patients and clients. Qualified practitioners are registered through the NMC and the NMC has the right to suspend or remove practitioners from the register if it is proven that the practitioner is not safe, or does not behave in a professional manner.

The NMC also sets out guidelines and criteria for education and practice, gives advice to nurses, midwives and specialist community public health nurses, and publishes numerous publications to support good practice.

Among the NMC publications you will find most useful are the:

- ● *Code of professional conduct: standards for conduct, performance and ethics*
- ● *Guidelines for records and record keeping*
- ● *Guidelines for the administration of medication.*

These publications are important but they are also fluid and are updated regularly. They are available free – either on the NMC website or by post on request. You can search the NMC website for information on many different subjects and most of the NMC publications are available on the NMC website as a document file.

Before the NMC, the United Kingdom Central Council (UKCC) had this responsibility. National Boards in each of the four countries of the United Kingdom worked with the UKCC: these National Boards were disbanded and, together with the UKCC, they became the NMC in 2002.

The NMC is accessible to practitioners and members of the public:

- Postal address: Nursing and Midwifery Council, 23 Portland Place, London W1B 1PZ
- Web address: http://www.nmc-uk.org
- Telephone enquiries: main switchboard: 020 7637 7181; registrations: 020 7333 9333; overseas application: 020 7333 6000; employers: 020 7631 3200; fitness to practise: 020 7333 6564; professional advice: 020 7333 6550; press enquiries: 020 7333 6557/6558.

Being a qualified nurse is a huge responsibility but the NMC has provided resources to help you. This chapter looks at those resources and how they support you in the responsible, competent and safe practice of professional nursing.

Throughout the chapter, I will refer to 'patients' and 'nurses'. I am using these as general terms for clarity – for ease of reading – and not in any way to minimise or exclude any individual or group of professionals or members of the public.

Although the NMC *Code of professional conduct* is the most commonly cited, *all* of the NMC guidance is intended to lead your professional practice. The directives all work together. Use the other directives to help you understand your obligations under the *Code of professional conduct*.

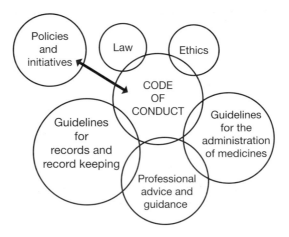

OBLIGATIONS AND EXPECTATIONS OF THE PROFESSIONAL NURSE: THE NMC *CODE OF PROFESSIONAL CONDUCT*

The *Code of professional conduct* contains guidelines for the expectations the NMC has for you as a nurse. No matter how it's written, those guidelines will be the same:

- You are accountable for your practice and responsible for what happens to people for whom you care.
- You must work cooperatively with others, be they other professionals, informal carers, patients – anyone with whom you come in contact in your daily work.
- You must protect patients, through following laws such as those pertaining to confidentiality, consent and the protection of vulnerable people, as well as through health and safety practices and through good nursing practice.
- Part of protecting patients is making sure your knowledge and skills are up to date.
- You must be the kind of nurse that people – patients, the public and other professionals – can look up to with respect. If you are not, patients will not be able to trust you and this will adversely affect the special, privileged relationship you have with them.
- You should identify when patients and others are at risk. It is not enough to help someone get better, you should – when possible – prevent them from becoming ill in the first place. This can be through education, care planning or just by having a good talk with someone when they need it.

The *Code of professional conduct* is there to explain what nurses do, in the hope that all nurses will live up to the expectations knowing that if they don't, the NMC has the power to prevent them from practising as nurses. It sets a precedent and the ground rules. Basically, it outlines:

- The standard of practice and conduct expected of you as a professional nurse.
- What members of the public should be able to expect of a nurse, midwife or health visitor.

In plain English, the *Code of professional conduct* says:

"Everything you do as a nurse – the way you work with others, the
way you behave and communicate, every action you take – should
be done with the best interest of your patient in mind."

As a nurse, the NMC gives you one guiding principle: You must be the kind of person who is able, in practice as a nurse, to put the patient first.

Respect the patient or client as an individual

It is your duty to make certain that the people for whom you are caring are treated with respect and dignity, and are given choices and opportunities to express their own opinions and decisions about their life and their care.

Everyone, but especially vulnerable people, has the right to be treated fully and wholly as a person. No one person is greater or more deserving than any other. Age, race, gender, religion, sexual orientation, lifestyle, culture, social or economic status, political beliefs, physical or mental disability – it doesn't matter. Every individual is equally precious and valuable. Your role doesn't stop with just acting for yourself, in your own practice. The *Code of professional conduct* says you must 'promote and protect the interests and dignity of patients . . .'. This might mean speaking up for a group of people by challenging protocols or practices. We must respect our patients and make sure others do as well. This could mean challenging the lack of information for a certain group, or that the criteria for a particular service unfairly discriminate against a group.

Respecting individuality means letting people make decisions for themselves. You have an obligation to provide people with information about health and social care and how to access care and support, but you can't make decisions for people as long as they are competent to make those decisions for themselves. It doesn't matter if you agree or if you think that they might have a better quality of life if they do what you tell them. Part of being a nurse is recognising that people have the right to live the life they want, as the *Code of professional conduct* says, 'within the limits of professional practice, existing legislation, resources and the goals of the therapeutic relationship'.

Respecting people also means having boundaries. You also can't ever exploit your role as a nurse – you can't use the fact you are caring for someone to gain at their expense. That gain might be physical, social or economic – no matter how, it's wrong. Benefiting at a patient's expense is abuse, because your job is to take care of people, not have them take care of you.

Obtain consent before you give any treatment or care

The *Code of professional conduct* states:
"*When obtaining valid consent, you must be sure that it is:*

- *given by a legally competent person*
- *given voluntarily*
- *informed.*"

Every person is legally competent unless a 'suitably qualified practitioner' decides that they are not. Competence to make a decision can

vary depending on what the decision is: someone who is not competent to consent to heart surgery might be competent to decide they
don't want to take a bath. Being legally competent means the person
can understand what the treatment is, what the consequences are,
and make a conscious choice.

Consent (or lack of consent) can be given in writing, verbally or
simply by cooperating. A patient who hands you their arm when you
say 'Can I take your blood pressure' has given you consent. A patient
who won't drink something is refusing.

If it's an emergency and the patient can't tell you what he or she
wants, you are expected to do whatever is necessary to preserve life.
You can't use these circumstances to over-ride what you know the
patient would say if he or she was able. Sometimes individuals will
have left advice with family or friends, or left a document such as a
'preferred place of care' (a document that allows people to express
their wishes for end-of-life care) stipulating their wishes. You can look
at the patient's past history: if that person has said 'no' several times
to a procedure, you should know in your heart that, if you were able
to ask, he or she would probably still say 'No'. Several years ago there
was a story in the news about a hospital near my home in America. A
patient who had a religious objection to a blood transfusion was in
A&E bleeding to death. The patient refused blood, even though he
knew this meant he would die. As soon as he became unconscious, a
doctor started a transfusion. Technically, this fitted the criteria – it was
an emergency and it was to preserve life – but the patient clearly had
competently refused.

Consent also applies to people with mental health problems or
learning disabilities: these individuals still have the right to refuse and
consent to care. If someone is sectioned under the Mental Health Act,
or if the Courts have appointed someone designated to make decisions on behalf of the individual, it is expected that people who know
the patient would participate in the assessment and care/treatment
planning to make certain that the person's wishes are respected and
that care decisions are made in the individual's best interest.

With children, there are special considerations around competence
to consent. Parents can give (or refuse) consent, but the age and ability
of the child to understand are taken into consideration. If you are
working with children, you need to be aware of the specific protocols
and procedures around consent.

The truth is that, under law, no one (except, with certain limitations,
a parent or a Court-appointed guardian) automatically has the right
to make a decision on behalf of anyone else. You have to be sure as
much as it is possible that whatever you do is what the patient would
want.

Obtaining consent

Obtaining consent is more than just asking a person if something is OK. As a nurse, you must make sure that the patient understands what giving consent really means.

It also means making sure the patient is aware of alternatives and options. This isn't necessarily you speaking to the patient about those options, but it might mean you challenging someone else to make sure they have. As an example:

> You are a theatre nurse. Mrs Turland is about to have her anaesthesia. As you are helping her, she asks you a question about the procedure. You know that the question should have been answered as part of giving consent.

Did you know that you have an obligation to stop and make sure her question is fully answered before she has the procedure? Will that get people all hot and bothered? Probably. Will people feel that this is an avoidable delay? Probably. Should you just assume that she forgot, so that the procedure starts on time and no one gets upset? No, absolutely not. Your duty is to protect the patient and no obligation is more important. No one, not the greatest and mightiest consultant, not an MP, not even the ruling monarch, is more important than your patient.

All individuals have the right to information about their health and what is happening to them. We are obliged to provide information that is honest, accurate and presented in a way that makes it as easy as possible for the patient to understand.

Sometimes, patients' families might say 'Don't tell them'. It is true that some people might not want to know, or might want someone else to make decisions for them. If someone's family says 'Don't tell my mother she has cancer, she wouldn't want to know' you should be sensitive to the patient's wishes, but you need to know who has decided that the patient doesn't want to know. It might be as simple as asking the patient 'If there was something really wrong with your health, how much would you want us to tell you?'. If the patient says 'Talk to my daughter about that . . .' you have your answer. If the patient says 'Tell me everything; I want to know it all . . .' then this is a very difficult situation: you need to seek advice from your employer, from the NMC, from a solicitor or from your union/professional organisation.

Part of consenting is respecting when patients say 'No'. As long as you are sure the patient understands the consequences, then that person has the right to say 'No', even if refusal shortens his or her life. Only a Court can force someone to have treatment. This is a legal right: it differs only when the health of an unborn child is at stake, when the team would need to look at the situation and make a decision about what to do.

The truth is that, under law, no one (except a parent, with certain limitations) automatically has the right to make a decision on behalf of anyone else.

Think about this: does an elderly person who won't take his heart tablet have the right not to take it? Do you have the right to hide it in food to make him take it?

Documentation

The person who 'gets' a patient's consent must document it. This can be by adding a document the patient has signed to the patient record, or writing something like 'Explained intubation and ventilation procedure to patient. Explained possible risks and likely outcomes. Patient stated that the procedure should go ahead. Patient unable to sign document due to physical condition. Consent witnessed by nurse V Tremayne'.

If consent should have been documented but isn't, you must make sure that someone actually did ensure that the patient gave consent. An example of this is when a patient hasn't signed a consent form for surgery. You shouldn't just say 'Sign this'. You should ask the person responsible for the surgery to come and make sure the patient gives consent. You might not be able to determine that the patient truly is consenting because you might not understand the risks or have the information the patient needs to make an informed choice.

You should also document any refusal:

> Attempted to give Mr Patterson an injection of insulin. Mr Patterson stated 'I don't want that any more' and put his hands up in a 'Stop' position. I explained the importance of insulin and what could happen if he didn't have the injection. Mr Patterson said 'I don't care if I go blind or my kidneys fail – I'm not having any more needles'. Mr Patterson is oriented to person, place and time, and does not appear confused. No history of dementia or confusion. Referred to Diabetes Specialist Nurse for further assessment. Insulin not given. Doctor made aware.

In the above example, the nurse doesn't just say 'He said "No", I said "OK"'. The nurse shows that she is making sure the patient has the support and help he needs, by documenting that she referred him to the Diabetes Nurse. She is also documenting that the person was not confused; this shows that she did check to see if the patient was competent.

Think about this: if Mr Patterson went into a coma, would you then give him the insulin?

Act to identify and minimise risk to patients and clients

Everything you do – or fail to do – is your responsibility. You can't blame anyone else – there is no get-out clause that you were 'only following orders'. As a nurse, you have an obligation always to act in the best interest of the people for whom you care. This could mean telling a colleague or another professional that he or she is wrong. Again, your patients have to trust that everything you do is always in their best interest. It's your duty to make sure your patients are safe and that their care is appropriate and delivered competently.

You must make sure that your practice, the care you deliver and the environment in which it is delivered are safe, therapeutic and ethical. If you believe a patient to be at risk, because you are concerned that for whatever reason another practitioner might not be fit to practise, you are obliged to speak up. If you are concerned about doing this, contact the NMC, your union/trade organisation or speak to your manager. All organisations have policies in place to guide your actions. Remember: the patient comes first.

When it comes to patients being at risk, you can't afford to wait: if you are worried that a patient is at risk because of the environment and you can't fix it yourself, you *must* report your concerns to someone senior. It must also be in writing. That's where incident reports come from!

Because you are a nurse 24 hours a day, on or off duty, you have a duty to provide care even when you are not at work. You don't have to be a paramedic – what you need to do is act reasonably to prevent the person from coming to further harm. If you are a mental health nurse and you arrive at the scene of a traffic accident, all that might be expected of you would be to move the injured person into the recovery position; if you were an experienced A&E nurse, a little more might be expected! The NMC says 'The care provided would be judged against what could reasonably be expected from someone with your knowledge, skills and abilities when placed in those particular circum-stances'. What you can't do is walk past as if nothing happened. For example:

> You are working on a very busy surgical ward. All the beds are full; the hospital is at full capacity. You find that one of the nurse call lights is broken; no matter what you do you can't get it to work. There isn't another bed to move the patient into. What do you do?

Think about this: Harold Shipman changed the world when he took such cruel advantage of his patients. Now we need to be more careful than ever, not only with the drugs we give and how we document our care (which is what the results of the Shipman enquiry means to most people) but also by becoming critical thinkers.

How many people have since reflected that they thought it was odd that Dr Shipman used so much morphine, and that so many more of his patients died at home in relation to similar-sized practices? People later said they had doubts. Why did no-one to speak out? What was it that kept them silent?

If someone had raised these concerns, there might be quite a few people around today living useful, happy lives. If you think something is not right, reflect on it. If you have nagging doubts, raise your concerns. I am sure that the people who didn't speak up about their concerns over Dr Shipman have trouble sleeping at night, realising how much they could have done by speaking up. It's not a lesson to learn in hindsight.

If you are worried someone will get angry at you for raising your concerns, think of the consequences if you don't. Who would you rather face, a colleague annoyed with you for a few days or a coroner asking why you didn't raise your concerns with someone?

Competency and trust
This is one area where post-registration education and practice (PREP) comes in (see Chapter 10 for more information on PREP) – by providing evidence that you are maintaining your professional competency, you are helping to reassure the public that nurses are competent and knowledgeable. If members of the public trust that we are competent, and that they can trust our care and our advice, they will come to us for help.

Another area that you have to think about is what happens if you find that for some reason you simply can't participate in someone's care?

An example could be a termination of a pregnancy. Perhaps you don't believe in terminations; that doesn't mean you can just abandon the patient to her own devices. If you find that you can't care for someone, you have to find someone who will take care of them. You have an obligation to try to avoid circumstances where your personal beliefs might conflict with the patient's beliefs or rights.

Think about this: You need to get home for an appointment. The nurse who is replacing you is late. Because this is a small nursing home, you are the only nurse. Can you leave before the other nurse gets there?

Cooperate with others in the team

You have to work with many other people: nurses, midwives, other clinicians, social workers, people from voluntary agencies, people from government organisations, universities . . . the list of professionals who you might come in contact with during your work is endless. In addition to the 'professional' team, you should also consider the patient and their family and carers as part of the overall team.

You need to remember that everyone has their opinion and contribution to make. You should make it easy for people to work together, in the patient's best interest, by communication and by sharing your own knowledge and skill.

An essential part of communication is the written record. Often, when you are working with people in a team, the only way you know them is by their handwriting in the patient's record. Your records should be accurate and written in a timely manner, and should 'provide clear evidence of the care planned, the decisions made, the care delivered and the information shared'.

Just because you are a member of a team doesn't mean that the team shares accountability for all decisions and actions: each professional is personally accountable for the decisions he or she makes and the actions he or she takes (or fails to take). In addition, as a nurse you are accountable for any tasks you delegate to other team members. You have to be certain you delegate appropriately and safely.

As a nurse, you should also remember that students are part of the team, and you have an obligation to facilitate their learning (there is more on mentorship in Chapter 7).

Think about this: If someone with more authority than you tells you to do something, but you don't think you should, can you say no?

Maintain your professional knowledge and competence

As a nurse, you are required to maintain your knowledge and skill. You have to take part in activities that help you learn, and keep your skills up to date (see the section on evidence-based practice in Chapter 4).

You not only need to know what to do, you need to know what you are *not* competent to do. As a professional, you have to be willing to say 'I am not good enough to be able to do that'. This is part of keeping your patients safe and being worthy of their trust.

If you realise that your skills are lacking, it's up to you to get help to improve your skills. The knowledge and skills framework (KSF; see Chapter 10) is designed to help you identify the skills and knowledge you need. Speak to your manager to sort out how you can develop in areas you aren't confident.

Remember that you should base your care on appropriate evidence and research. Evidence-based practice (see Chapter 4) is key to showing that you are a thoughtful, safe and competent practitioner.

Think about this: You have seen someone insert an intravenous cannula many times. You took a training course 2 years ago. A patient needs an IV now. The patient's veins look good and you think you might be able to get it in. What do you do?

Be trustworthy

Trust is about making sure the people you care for will allow you to care for them. For that to happen, they must trust that you:

- Are worthy of their trust: people for whom we care allow us an intimacy that is usually reserved for family members. We touch them, talk to them about very sensitive and personal things, and we have access to privileged information.
- Are honest and will not take advantage of your privileged relationship.
- Will help them as individuals and as members of a community to have the healthiest life possible, no matter their limitations or the choices they might make in their life. Why should they come to us if we aren't going to help?
- Will make decisions based not on any kind of personal gain but only for the best interests of your patients.

Patients must also have faith that nurses are trustworthy professionals who will act professionally and in accordance with law and ethical principles: as a nurse, everything you do reflects on nurses and nursing. When the NMC *Code of professional conduct* speaks about 'uphold and enhance the good reputation of the professions', what it is really saying is that you have to accept that they way you behave could influence the way the public thinks and feels about nurses. If you break a law – for example, if you were arrested for stealing – how could anyone trust you? Might they think that all nurses were potentially thieves? If you wear your uniform in public, could it make people worried about your uniform carrying an infection? That could make them worry about loved ones in hospital, or might prevent them from seeking help for themselves.

Members of the public must also trust that you will keep their information confidential. You must follow the Data Protection Act, but go even further – everything you do should shield the patient from unnecessary embarrassment or exposure. From draping the patient during a procedure, to not gossiping about patients, to making certain you protect patient records, it is your job to keep private things private. People who don't have a right to know, or see, information about a patient shouldn't be able to. You should let patients know that you won't share information about them without asking them first. This includes telling families and friends!

The exception to divulging information without express consent is when vulnerable people are at risk (for example, from child or elder abuse), if there is a genuine concern about someone being at risk of significant harm or if you are required by law or a Court order to do so. If you are unsure, you should seek support from the NMC, your union/professional organisation, or someone at your place of work. Every Trust/healthcare workplace has policies about confidentiality and disclosure of information.

One final thing about trust is that to make sure you are never motivated by personal gain, the NMC *Code of professional conduct* specifically forbids you from using your role as a nurse to endorse any commercial product or service, and from accepting gifts or loans from patients, their families or friends. There is a difference between accepting a box of chocolates for the entire ward when a patient is discharged and accepting a £20 note from a patient for whom you are currently caring. In no way should it ever seem that the patient has to bribe or tip you to get care. Your motives must always remain absolutely above question. For example:

> You are caring for a young man, Erique, who has learning disabilities. He has been poorly. A man telephones to ask how Erique is; he tells you he is Erique's brother. You can't find any information in your client's notes about family members. What do you do?

Indemnity insurance

The final section of the NMC *Code of professional conduct* is about indemnity insurance. It recommends that every practitioner covered by the NMC has professional indemnity insurance to cover in case of an allegation of professional negligence, either at or outside work.

Although your employer might provide some coverage, it's up to you to make sure that you have adequate coverage. Unions and professional organisations often offer indemnity insurance as part of their membership benefits.

DOCUMENTATION AND THE GUIDELINES FOR RECORDS AND RECORD KEEPING

You have a legal and professional obligation to make sure you keep accurate, appropriate clinical records. The NMC has excellent guidelines about how records should be kept. Although those guidelines are explicit in the *Guidelines for records and record keeping*, they are also implicit in the NMC *Code of professional conduct*.

Why keep good records? Remember the principles of the *Code of professional conduct*:

- respect the patient or client as an individual
- obtain consent before you give any treatment or care
- protect confidential information
- cooperate with others in the team
- maintain your professional knowledge and competence
- be trustworthy
- act to identify and minimise risk to patients and clients.

Your record keeping should show that you are meeting your obligations under the *Code of professional conduct*:

- Good record keeping is respectful and shows that you have treated the patient as an individual.
- Documentation that the patient consents, perhaps even simply by participating in care, proves that you are aware that the patient should consent to all care and treatment.
- Managing documentation properly is one part of protecting confidential information.
- Communication, through written documentation, is key to cooperative multidisciplinary team working.
- Good record keeping, including specialised documents such as care planning and assessments, show that you are delivering evidence-based, competent care.
- By keeping good records you are showing that you are worthy of the trust placed in you for the care of your patients.
- Good record keeping and documentation will identify and plan to minimise risks for patients.

If you fail to keep proper documentation, you are failing the *Code of professional conduct*. It is that simple. There are some key points to remember when writing things in patient notes:

- Notes must be made in a timely manner. If something significant happens, write it down as soon as possible afterwards. Notes should be in a chronological consecutive order. This means you should date and time each entry.
- Don't use abbreviations, except that when the abbreviation will be absolutely perfectly clear to any other reader, even one that is not a healthcare professional.

- Don't use slang or jargon.
- Write with a black, non-erasable pen.
- Never use Tippex™. If you must correct an error, put a single line through it, write 'error' above it, initial it and carry on. If you write an entry in the wrong patient's notes, cross through it, make another entry below it that says 'The above was entered incorrectly into the wrong patient's notes' and sign it.
- Be clear and specific: don't write 'Patient in pain. Given meds.' Write 'At 10.00 a.m. patient complained of pain in the surgical area on a scale of 6/10. Given 10 mg of morphine orally at 10.20 a.m. At 11.00 a.m. patient said pain was much better and said no further medication was needed'. Write exactly what you did and when. You might be criticised for writing long notes but, legally, writing clear and specific notes is correct.
- Be objective and non-judgemental: write your notes as if the person you are writing about is going to be reading them while sitting next to his or her solicitor. If you want to convey how someone is acting, simply repeat word for word what he or she tells you. Don't say someone is aggressive or violent. Say 'Patient states "I am going to throw this at you if you come any closer!" '. If the patient swears, repeat the swear words exactly. This says everything someone else needs to know without you being accused of making a judgement. Don't write 'Patient was angry'; write 'Patient didn't make eye contact, had arms across chest, brows furrowed and was pacing . . .'. Describe what you see and what you hear, and let anyone else reading it make up their own mind!
- Don't leave blank areas for other people to fill things in. Put a line through all empty space, and clearly sign your name at the end of your note. Do not leave a blank space before or after your documentation.
- Print your name and title along with your signature unless there is a signature sheet in the record.

Here are some examples of poor record keeping:

| 26/5/05 11.30 a.m. | Mr. Ponga is argumentative and impossible; he won't wash and he won't allow anyone to wash him. |

What's wrong? This note is judgemental. Look at the note below; it puts the point across without making the person look bad:

| 26/5/05
11.30 a.m. | Mr. Ponga requires strong encouragement to complete personal hygiene. He states 'I'm not doing it - leave me alone!'. Mr. Ponga is physically able to complete personal care tasks independently. Late staff will be asked to offer Mr. Ponga a bath as he hasn't washed this morning. |

Try this next one – what is this nurse really saying?

| 8/8/05
8.00 a.m. | Slept well. Catheter draining. Bowels open. No complaints. |

Slept well? For how long. Catheter draining . . . what? What colour urine? How much? The note says nothing about the patient's condition or the night the patient had. It looks like it should, but it doesn't say anything at all. Compare it with this note:

| 8/8/05
8.00 a.m. | Mrs. Jalanni slept from about 10pm until 6am. Urinary catheter care done; catheter drained appx 600 ml clear yellow urine; no obvious sediment or debris. Patient declined pain medication stating 'I feel OK in myself'. At 6 a.m. patient opened bowels, large amount Bristol Stool 5. |

Is this note more helpful to the team, and to the patient's overall care, than the first one?

Here is another note: what do you think of this one?

| 7/2/05 | Patient should have had incontinence assessment this morning but it was left for evening staff. It's not fair that days left this for us because we are busy enough. Patient has stress incontinence only. |

The patient record is not the place to air differences with staff. If it doesn't relate to the patient or the patient's care, it doesn't belong in the notes. Full stop. This type of entry is highly unprofessional.

Here is an entry you might find in a community patient's notes:

| 21/5/05 | Care per plan. |

This note says nothing except 'I was here'. What care? What care plan? This might be a better option:

| 21/5/05 | Wound dressing changed per care plan 1. Assessment recorded on Wound Care worksheet. Wound remains very sore and red. Have swabbed and counselled patient to continue taking antibiotics as ordered. |

The note above shows that you actually assessed the wound and spoke to the patient.

Now try this example:

| 3/11/05 | Pt in w/c × 2 h am. Amb × 2 m w/ OT w/ RF. TC > Onco Cons– pt OP appt 1/12. Sr Bilston book Tx. Pt c/o +++ pain /p amb. Med given. |

What? Some of the abbreviations could be misinterpreted. Some of them were not clear, and some really didn't explain anything (+++ pain? What's that?). Write notes in clear language.

| 3/11/05 | Patient in wheelchair for 2 hours this morning. Walked 2 metres with rolling frame with OT. Call from Oncologist: pt will have Outpatient 1 month; Sr Bilston has booked transport. Pt complained of significant pain after ambulation: 7 on scale of 1–10. Given paracetamol 1000 mg; patient reports pain relieved. |

This last example is the worst note of all:

| 14/10/05 | Doliiml vos luuml im rizqvrotary blsless . . . |

If you can't write legibly, then **print**. Your notes might as well not even be there if no one can read them. Also, errors can be made as a result of poor or illegible writing. I know a doctor who once who wrote 'methotrexate 75 mg'. Well, that's what it looked like – the actual dose was 7.5 mg but his handwriting was bad and it was difficult to see the "." in '7.5' mg. Because it was a specialist chemotherapy unit, strange doses were common and often went unquestioned. The nurse was about to administer the dose when a nursing student decided to question it with the pharmacist, who held the dose until the doctor was contacted to confirm the order. The doctor literally broke into a sweat when he realised how the order had been mis-interpreted: for that patient, the dose would probably have been fatal. If the patient had received the dose, it would have been the nurse's error: ultimately, when you administer a medication, it's your responsibility to make sure you are giving the right medication in the right dose.

This gives rise to another issue about documentation: it's not just your documentation you have to worry about: you have to challenge documentation that is illegible. It's not enough to look at some hiero-glyphic hen-scratches and say 'Ooh, I really am pretty sure it says . . .'; you have to be certain. If that means calling another person and saying, 'Can you come back and write this so we can read it?' then that's what you need to do.

Your notes are the direct reflection of your knowledge, skill and competency, and poor record keeping could raise questions about your competence under the NMC *Code of professional conduct*.

MEDICATION ADMINISTRATION AND THE GUIDELINES FOR THE ADMINISTRATION OF MEDICATIONS

The incident about the methotrexate described above highlights how good documentation and appropriate medication administration go hand in hand. In nursing, nothing is really an isolated skill. Medication administration, seen as a central nursing role, is potentially a risky intervention and should be approached carefully and critically each and every time it is carried out. Complacency is dangerous. The NMC says:

> "The administration of medicines is an important aspect of the professional practice of persons whose names are on the Council's register. It is not solely a mechanistic task to be performed in strict compliance with the written prescription of a medical practitioner. It requires thought and the exercise of professional judgement . . . "

You have a number of obligations when you administer medication:

1. The six rights:

- give the **right medication,**
- in the **right dose** and
- through the **right route,**
- to the **right patient,**
- at the **right time** and
- with the **right documentation**.

There is more on the six rights later in this section.

2. Know what the medication is for, and know likely side effects or contraindications:

- This isn't about knowing real gutsy pharmacodynamics – you need to know how the medication you are about to put into your patient will affect that person and how that will impact your care. For example, you need to know that digoxin slows the heart rate and that morphine causes respiratory depression.
- You have to know enough about what the drug will do so that you can know if you need to withhold it or notify the prescriber of an adverse reaction.

3. Educate the patient about the medication whenever possible:

- Individuals who understand the reasons they take medications are more likely to feel in control of their care and treatment. Would you want to take something if you weren't sure what it did?
- In addition to education about specific medications, it is important to educate patients and their carers about general medication issues: storage, finishing medications when prescribed, not sharing medications, etc.

4. Make sure that medications are properly stored and protected:

- Controlled drugs must be secure; drugs should be stored at the correct temperature, etc.
- Patients and their carers should understand about the storage and care of medications.

5. Make sure that you know the special risks for the group of patients you care for:

- Age, infirmity and various illnesses can affect the actions of medication.
- Drug dosages vary in different patient groups.
- Certain drugs can be used for one reason in one group of clients and differently in another.

- Some groups, such as older people, may have a significant number of medications. Having many different medications, called poly-pharmacy, puts patients at significant risk.

All in all, when you give medications, you must be absolutely confident that patients:

- are getting what the prescriber intended them to get, the way the prescriber intended them to get it
- are safe in receiving the medication
- understand what they are receiving and why
- understand how to take and how to store their medication
- understand and can recognise potential side effects, and know what to do if they occur
- have given their consent.

Considering everything you know about medication administration, let's look once more at the 'six rights':

- **Give the right medication:** an appropriate medication for this patient, considering the patient's particular needs and circumstances. For example:

> If a patient is vegan and you are directed to apply a dressing made from pork, is this the right medication? Did you realise that dressings can be considered medications?

- **In the right dose:** an appropriately calculated dose for this patient, considering their individual circumstances and needs. For example:

> If you are not certain if the dosage is correct, how could you challenge it?

- **Through the right route:** an appropriate route for this patient, considering the patient's particular needs and circumstances. For example:

> If all the medications for a patient who is vomiting are oral, do you give them, hold them, or call the prescriber and ask for an alternative route?

- **To the right patient:** correctly identify beyond any doubt that the patient for whom the medication is prescribed is the patient to whom you are giving the medication. For example:

> If the patient doesn't have any identification, how can you be certain that you have the right patient? If you ask the patient her name, would you say 'Are you Mrs Howarth?' or 'What is your name please?' (Hint: it's easier to make a mistake by asking 'Are you Mrs Howarth?' because the answer is limited to 'Yes', 'No' or 'I don't know'.)

- **At the right time:** the right time for this patient, considering his or her individual circumstances and needs, and considering the availability of an appropriate person to administer or assist the patient in administering the medication. For example:

> If your patient has to take a tablet four times a day, is this four times during waking hours (7 a.m., midday, 5 p.m., 10 p.m.) or every 6 hours around the clock (7 a.m., 1 p.m., 7 p.m., 1 a.m.)? Is it reasonable to expect someone to wake up at 1 a.m. to take a medication? If the patient needs District Nurse assistance to administer eye drops, is it wise to schedule them for 6 a.m.?

- **With correct documentation:**

> Is it just your documentation that matters? If you crush a tablet, how and where do you document that? What if you don't sign off the medication record? If it's not written, was it done? How could that affect the patient?

A final note about medication administration: you need to be certain that your drug calculations and maths skills are flawless. Use a calculator, double-check with others but always make sure you have calculated appropriately. If your maths skills are poor, your employer has an obligation to help you – but they can't help you if you don't tell them you need help. Eventually, when you make a drug error, they will find out anyway.

Drug calculations

If you need to improve your drug calculations and maths skills, I strongly suggest you get a book like *Nursing calculations* by John

Gatford and Nicole Phillips. It covers all the basics and will give you valuable practice. This section provides a basic review of numeracy: conversions and calculations.

Basic conversions

Basic numeracy is essential for nurses. Even if you are OK with the basics, keep a calculator handy and consider double-checking your calculations with another nurse.

Basic measurements

Table 9.1

Name of unit	Symbol	What it measures
Metre	m	Length
Gram	gm or g	Mass
Litre	L	Fluid

There are other units of measurement:

Table 9.2

1000 units	Unit	1/100 units	1/1000 units	1/1 000 000 units
Kilometre	Metre (m)	Centimetre (cm)	Millimetre (mm)	
Kilolitre	Litre (L)	Centilitre (cL)	Millilitre (mL)	
Kilogram	Gram (g)	Centigram	Milligram (mg)	Microgram (mcg)

You must always be careful with abbreviations: write out the entire unit. Don't write 'mcg,' write 'microgram': 'mcg' can look like 'mg' – and there is a huge difference in the amount.

Also, you need to be adept with the metric system. The basics of metric conversions are:

- To convert from a larger unit to a smaller one, the decimal moves to the right.
- To convert from a smaller unit to a larger one, the decimal point moves left.
- You move the decimal point a number of places based on the difference between the units. It's usually three places.

You must be comfortable changing between different metric units. You also need to get comfortable with changing in between metric and Imperial measurements.

Table 9.3

Metric		Imperial
1 millimetre (mm)		0.03937 inches
1 centimetre (cm)	10 mm	0.3937 inches
1 metre (m)	100 cm	1.0936 yards

Table 9.4

Imperial		Metric
1 inch (in)		2.54 cm
1 foot (ft)	12 in	0.3048 m
1 yard (yd)	3 ft	0.9144 m

Table 9.5

Metric		Imperial
1 cubic metre (m^3)	1000 dm^3	1.3080 yd^3
1 litre (L)	1000 mL	1.76 pints
1 cubic centimetre (cm^3)		0.0610 in^3

Table 9.6

Imperial		Metric
1 cubic inch (in^3)		16.387 cm^3
1 cubic foot (ft^3)	1728 in^3	0.0283 m^3
1 fluid ounce (fl oz)		28.413 mL
1 pint (pt)	20 fl oz	0.5683 L
1 gallon (gal)	8 pt	4.5461 L

Remember: if you are using a US-based reference book, some measurements will differ (for example, there are 16 oz in a US pint).

Table 9.7

Metric		Imperial
1 milligram (mg)		0.0154 grain
1 gram (g)	1000 mg	0.0353 oz
1 kilogram (kg)	1000 g	2.2046 lb
1 tonne (t)	1000 kg	0.9842 ton

Table 9.8

Imperial		Metric
1 ounce (oz)	437.5 grain	28.35 g
1 pound (lb)	16 oz	0.4536 kg
1 stone	14 lb	6.3503 kg
1 hundredweight (cwt)	112 lb	50.802 kg

Calculations will be based on one of the units of measurement: to be correct, you have to have all the factors in the same unit of measurement. The most common error is in converting one unit of measure to another.

Sometimes a medication must be titrated (to be calculated based on an individual) to body weight or to body surface area (e.g. 1 mg/kg).

You always have to be able to make calculations using the same unit of measurement. This means there will be times you have to convert between units. If you are unsure of your conversions, have someone else double-check. It is good practice for any nurse to have someone double-check a calculation anyway!

Children's nurses, and some nurses in specialist areas such as ITU, will use special types of formulae and calculations. The calculations here are basic: please use specialist resources for other formulae. The most basic calculation is:

$$\text{Dose} = \frac{\text{Dose needed}}{\text{Dose on hand}} \times \text{Dose unit}$$

OK, try this out: you have 500-milligram capsules (that is, your dose unit is a 500-mg capsule) and you need to give 1000 milligrams:

$$\text{Dose} = \frac{1000\,\text{mg}}{500\,\text{mg}} \times 500\text{-mg capsule}$$

Dose = Two 500-mg capsules

You need to make sure you have the same unit of measurement or this formula will not work.

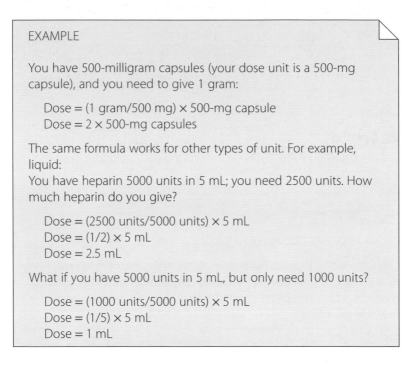

EXAMPLE

You have 500-milligram capsules (your dose unit is a 500-mg capsule), and you need to give 1 gram:

Dose = (1 gram/500 mg) × 500-mg capsule
Dose = 2 × 500-mg capsules

The same formula works for other types of unit. For example, liquid:
You have heparin 5000 units in 5 mL; you need 2500 units. How much heparin do you give?

Dose = (2500 units/5000 units) × 5 mL
Dose = (1/2) × 5 mL
Dose = 2.5 mL

What if you have 5000 units in 5 mL, but only need 1000 units?

Dose = (1000 units/5000 units) × 5 mL
Dose = (1/5) × 5 mL
Dose = 1 mL

This formula is very useful! There are others, but personally I find that having just one and being good at it works best.

Summary
- As a nurse, you are accountable for all your acts, or failures to act, irrespective of the direction, advice or orders of any other nurses or professional.
- You have obligations to your patients: to keep them safe, to respect them as unique individuals, to act to preserve and promote health both for the individual and for the community as a whole.
- You have to work with others: by working cooperatively, being a mentor/teacher and by challenging others to promote best practice in the patient's interest.
- Your acts and obligations are found not just in what you do, but how you document what you do.

- As a nurse, you must understand how to give medication appropriately: this includes understanding the medication and what it does, as well as making sure the dosage is properly calculated.
- In everything you do, you have an obligation to see the patient as an individual, and to work cooperatively with patient, carers and family to make certain that your care is in concordance with the patient's wishes and beliefs.
- You have an obligation as a nurse to always behave in a professional manner, in order to be worthy of trust and to uphold the good image and reputation of nurses and nursing: you are always a nurse, not just when you are at work.

Reference

Gatford J, Phillips N 2006 Nursing calculations. Churchill Livingstone, Edinburgh.

10 Personal development, planning and portfolios

- Personal development plans
- Post-registration education and practice
- The knowledge and skills framework
- Summary

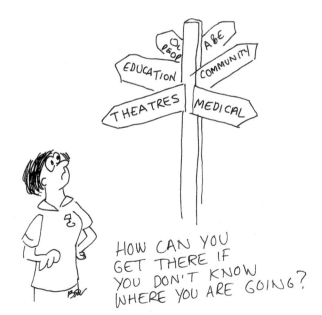

HOW CAN YOU GET THERE IF YOU DON'T KNOW WHERE YOU ARE GOING?

This chapter looks at your own personal and professional development. You will need to continue to prove over the course of your career that you have maintained your knowledge and competencies. You will also want to have a plan for growing into the kind of nurse you want to be. If you don't plan, you won't be ready when the opportunities you would like come up!

First, some definitions to make this a bit easier:

- **KSF: knowledge and skills framework:** under Agenda for Change, each job has a list of skills and knowledge that people in that job should have. The purpose of the KSF is to help you develop your knowledge and skill.
- **PDP: personal (or professional) development plan:** a plan through which you undertake to improve your knowledge and skill.
- **PPP: personal professional portfolio:** the portfolio of evidence that shows you have met your obligations under PREP.
- **PREP: post-registration education and practice:** the NMC requires that you show you have maintained fitness to practise in between your registration renewals.

PERSONAL DEVELOPMENT PLANS

Personal development plans (PDPs) help you identify and carry out development that you will need. The areas of development can be very diverse. You might want to develop in any of a number of areas, for example by:

- developing a new clinical skill
- developing knowledge of a disease or medical problem
- developing more assertiveness
- taking a certain specialty course
- gaining better II skills.

All of these things would be related to your practice as a nurse. The beauty of planning is that you can choose the areas you want to develop. As you probably have guessed, PDP and reflection are closely linked. As you reflect, you start to see what you need for development. The PDP then helps you work out *how* you are going to develop.

Some other areas that might drive your development planning are government initiatives and policies, which are:

- The National Service Frameworks, which require practitioners to give a certain level of care.
- Essence of Care, which outlines certain standards.
- The Department of Health, which puts out bulletins making recommendations about care and practice.
- The Knowledge and Skills Framework under Agenda for Change.

Your place of work will also offer training, courses and opportunities to further your education. Often, there are special initiatives to increase nursing knowledge or skill in certain areas.

The professional press (books and journals) can also help you become aware of areas where you need to develop. For example, you might have read an article about catheter care in the *Nursing Standard* or *Nursing Times*, and it made you realise that you don't have a good understanding of suprapubic catheterisations. You have recognised that this is a development need, as you care for patients with catheters.

In addition, there are national nursing forums, specialty nursing groups and organisations such as the Royal College of Nursing that will put out material designed to help you recognise gaps and advance your practice.

All of these things – reflection, policy, your employer, books and journals, and organisations – can give you ideas about how to develop your practice. They can also help you to develop that practice once you know what you want to do. But in order to get there, you need a plan.

The plan starts by you looking inward and taking an inventory of what you already know, what you can build on, what is weak and what you think you need.

Let's use Oliver as an example:

Oliver Thorpe is a new staff nurse on a ward for older people. He wants to become a clinical nurse specialist in a couple of years and perhaps do a Master's degree in advanced practice. He has done some reading and observed the skills his more experienced colleagues have. He sits down and makes a list of things he needs.

I need to learn about:
1. wound care – I don't know what half the dressings do, or when to use them!
2. leg ulcer diagnosis and care
3. community assessment in general
4. making referrals
5. evidence-based practice, research and audit.

Oliver has reflected on a number of things since he started in this post. He has identified that there are a few things he would like to improve:

1. *I need to be more assertive.*
2. *I need to improve my time management skills.*
3. *I need to learn more about the documentation used by my team.*

Finally, Oliver knows from his team leader that he will be expected to use a new form:

1. *I need to learn more about the single assessment process and SAP forms.*

As a new nurse, Oliver has identified nine areas in which he wants to develop himself and his practice. He decides to focus on just one area for now: wound care. Remember the nursing process (assess, plan, implement/intervention, evaluation) mentioned in Chapter 2? In the same way, Oliver has done his assessment and moves on to his plan.

The first step of the plan is actually a transition between your assessment and your plan. In the initial stage, you are looking more in-depth at each of your assessed needs. It has two real purposes: to help keep you motivated because you really understand why you need this level of development, and to help you think out what you need to do to achieve goals.

Your initial plan should be based on a basic formula.

What? Why? Where? When? How? and Who?

- **What** do I need to learn or do? What do I need for funding?
- **Why** is it important for me to do this?
- **Where** will I be once I have done this?
- **When** are the classes/in-service training held? How soon do I need to do this?
- **How** will I accomplish this and how much time will I need? (including a timeline for actions)
- **Who** can help me to achieve this? Who might pay for this course/in-service training?

Looking at his development needs for 'wound care', Oliver makes the following plan:

Table 10.1

What	Improve understanding of wound care and wound care products.	
Why	I need to make good decisions about wound care because it is integral to my role as a community nurse	
Where	Once I am more knowledgeable, I will be more confident, be more useful to my team and be able to provide better patient care	
When	I need to learn this soon, because a lot of what I already do requires this knowledge. I hope that within 3 months I will have an improved understanding of wound care products	
How	I will make an appointment to speak to the team leader to discuss my plan and ask for support.	To meet by 12 Jan
	I will contact training and development and find out about wound care courses	By 7 Jan
	Weekly for the next three months, I will review journal articles that discuss wound care and products	
	I will ask the district nurse to spend some time helping me learn	By 7 Jan
	Whenever it is appropriate, I will ask colleagues about the materials they are using	
	I will call Tissue Viability and ask about courses and information	By 12 Jan
	I would like to take the Degree level Wound Care Course at University of Middle Earth (UME)	To be enrolled by 27 October
Who	District Nurse/ team leader Tissue viability Other team members Training and development staff	

Oliver is confident that this is a good basic plan. However, after speaking to his team leader, he also realises that 'wound care' is a much bigger topic than he realised. He and his team leader make a further list:

- aetiology of wounds: acute and chronic wounds
- anatomy and physiology of wounds and healing
- wound-bed preparation

- classes of wound-care product
- wound-care techniques.

For each of these, he develops another plan:

Table 10.2

What	Understand the aetiology of wounds
Why	If I understand how wounds begin, I can help to prevent them and will understand what caused them in order to help them heal more quickly.
Where	My assessment of potential risks, and patient education will improve. By understanding the nature of the wound, I will be better able to choose the correct wound care product.
When	This is the first step to improving my understanding of wound care, so it must be done soon.
How	I will read the book recommended by my Team Leader — By 23 Feb
	I will take the wound care course given by Tissue Viability — 3 March-14 March
	I will search the net for information on the aetiology of wounds — Ongoing
	I will do case studies on our current patients who have wounds that fall into different classes, as chosen by my team leader
Who	District Nurse/ team leader
	Tissue viability
	Other team members

One thing Oliver notices is that there isn't a lot of information available on wound care and wound-care products in the team's office, so he starts to build a team resource folder as he finds information for himself.

After he has taken the wound-care course, Oliver realises that his team could use an audit of the patients' wounds and the wound-care products being used. He asks his team leader for help and together they design an audit tool. He brings it to a team meeting and asks everyone to use it.

Once he has all the information for the audit, Oliver and his team leader look at the findings. He finds that although most nurses use products in the way suggested by Tissue Viability (as specified in the policies given out in the wound-care course), in a few cases the dressings used don't seem to make sense. The team leader reviews these cases and decides that a team update on wound care would be useful. Oliver is asked to prepare a brief presentation on his audit and the team leader offers help so that Oliver can do a presentation on what the results mean for the team.

In May, Oliver reflects on all he has learned and meets with his team leader. The team leader is pleased with his progress and mentions that the team's care has improved as a result of the audit. He agrees that the wound-care course at the University of Middle Earth would be very useful and approves Oliver's study leave request. The team leader helps him sort out the funding.

As part of his evaluation, Oliver put all his reflections, the certificate from the Tissue Viability course and the audit results in his PREP and KSF portfolios. He also looks back at the list of things he wanted to learn:

1. ~~wound care — I don't know what half the dressings do, or when to use them!~~
2. leg ulcer diagnosis and care
3. community assessment in general
4. making referrals
5. evidence-based practice, research and audit
6. I need to be more assertive
7. I need to improve my time management skills
8. ~~I need to learn more about the documentation used by my team~~
9. I need to learn more about the single assessment process and SAP forms.

He realises that although he chose to focus on wound care, the process of meeting that goal will also help him to learn about leg ulcers (on the university course) and has already taught him about how patients' wound are assessed, how referrals are made to Tissue Viability for pressure-relieving equipment and about audit. He recognises that the whole process has helped him to become more assertive. As a result of planning and preparing for the audit – and from trying to focus on too many areas in the beginning! – his team leader has helped him learn some valuable time-management skills.

Oliver knows that his needs have changed, so he re-writes his list:

I need to develop my skills in the following areas:
1. To do and interpret Doppler examinations
2. To do a competent diabetic foot assessment.

From there, the process goes on . . . assessment, plan, intervention, evaluation. As he becomes stronger and more competent, Oliver might realise that instead of becoming a clinical nurse specialist for older people, he would rather become a Tissue Viability specialist. He might have found that wound care fascinates him and that he would like to help other nurses become stronger in that area.

He could, however, have spent two or three years as a staff nurse without a plan, taken in-services that seemed interesting, learned things as the opportunities arose. The result would have been:

- The team might not have developed a wound-care resource folder.
- There might not have been an audit.
- The care improvement from the audit might not have happened.
- Oliver might not have got onto the university course.
- Oliver might not have gained all the skills he did as a result of following his plan.
- Oliver might still be a junior staff nurse without a plan for his future career instead of preparing to become a Tissue Viability specialist nurse.

Oliver has benefited from his plan both as a person and as a professional. That is the real reason that PDP is valuable – it can be so much more than just a paperwork exercise – it can be a map to build your skills and career and help you find the place you really want to be.

Your personal development can be very simple – a staff nurse taking the time to learn first aid, for example, or very complex – a specialist nurse taking a Master's degree course. It doesn't matter – what's important is that you know what you want to achieve and that you develop a plan to achieve it.

There are many different ways to plan your personal development and the knowledge and skills framework will help highlight the things you need to know and be able to do in your work. Ultimately, however, as a nurse it's your career; you will enjoy it much more if you feel like you are learning and becoming the nurse you really want to be.

POST-REGISTRATION EDUCATION AND PRACTICE

Post-registration education and practice (PREP) links very nicely to PDP. As you saw with Oliver, what you do through PDP you can bring into your personal professional profile (PPP). Try to see it as PDP being the plan to meet your PREP, and your PPP being the place you store the results.

However, there is more to PREP than just filing your certificates and results. It should be a resource for you as you go through your career. According to the NMC's *PREP handbook* (available from the NMC on their website or by post) PREP helps you to:

- keep up to date with new developments in practice
- think and reflect for yourself
- demonstrate that you are keeping up to date and developing your practice
- provide the best possible care for your patients and clients.

Your portfolio

One common misconception is that there is one 'right' pattern for your portfolio. Although there are some common areas you will want to cover, what you do with the portfolio is really up to you. It's yours. As long as it meets the NMC criteria to prove you have met the requirements for renewing your registration , you can do with it whatever you like.

For example, you know that reflection is an important part of PREP. Perhaps you are not comfortable reflecting in your portfolio and would like to keep a separate reflective log. All you might need to put in your PPP is a summary of how reflection has changed you and your practice:

> Through reflection, I learned to improve my approach to
> elderly people with mental health problems, and on evaluation
> I have become a much more patient and sensitive practitioner . . .

You don't need to put the entire reflection if you don't want to. Just make sure you keep the original reflection someplace, in case the NMC ever wants to see it. Be honest with yourself in the reflection and don't worry about what other people might think when they read it. The purpose of PREP is to show that you are keeping your skills and knowledge up to date and that you are continuing to learn and grow as a nurse. The NMC gives you a basic outline for how you might frame learning activities in your portfolio. This is reprinted here:

PREP (CPD) PERIOD – the three year registration period to which this learning applies

From: to:

WORK PLACE – Where were you working when the learning activity took place?

Name of organisation:

Brief description of your work/role:

NATURE OF THE LEARNING ACTIVITY

Date:

Briefly describe the learning activity; for example, reading a relevant clinical article, attending a course, observing practice:

State how many hours this took:

DESCRIPTION OF THE LEARNING ACTIVITY –of what did it consist?

Describe what the learning activity consisted of – include for example: why you decided to do the learning activity or how the opportunity came about; where, when and how you did the learning activity; the type of learning activity: and what you expected to gain from it.

OUTCOME OF THE LEARNING ACTIVITY –How did the learning relate to your work?

Give a personal view of how the learning informed and influenced your work – what effect has this learning had on the way in which you work, or intend to work in the future? Do you have any ideas or plans for any follow-up learning?

The way in which this learning has influenced my work is . . .

There are some things you will always want to put in your PREP portfolio: your CV, certificates from training days (with the course outline or agenda so you have proof what the training entailed), any educational certificates. Certificates of attendance at conferences and events are good, too, but again make sure you have some information to show what you actually *did* at the event or conference.

If you have published an article, a review or even letters to the editor, save it for your PREP portfolio. Anything you do at or about work is potentially PREP material.

PREP isn't only about the things you do when on the job, you can also look at very creative ways to show that you are constantly learning as a nurse. Would you ever consider putting things like this in your portfolio?

> *Since becoming a mother myself, I have a much better understanding of how stressful it must be for a parent whose child is ill.*
>
> *When my grandmother died, I saw how important it was for the nurses caring for her to explain things and to prepare her in advance for the things she would need. This has helped me improve my patient education skills.*
>
> *That documentary about nurses undercover made me angry at first, then I realised that sometimes it is exactly the way the documentary showed it. I try to remember every day how terrible it would be if I acted as a nurse in the way I saw others acting. It helps keep me focused.*

So you see that you can use many different events and activities for your portfolio.

Here is a list of common subject headings that you may want to have in your PPP:

- **Personal information:** name, address, qualification, telephone, etc.
- **Work experience:** your most recent CV (see Chapter 2).
- **Education:** information about any diplomas, certificates and degrees you have achieved.
- **Training:** a list of in-services, trainings and courses, with dates and details of what you learned.
- **Reflections:** reflections and/or a summary of reflections.
- **Learning activities:** any 'alternative learning' you have done, for example, you watched a fascinating television show on anatomy where a person was actually autopsied and it helped you

understand more about digestion and problems with the digestive tract.
- **Testimonials:** any 'testimonials' – your appraisal, any letters from patients/families, from your employer, etc.

Your PPP will need to be around for a while, so make sure it meets the following:

- It has to be durable: although a paper or card folder is acceptable, a heavy-duty plastic folder might be better.
- It has to be serviceable: try using dividers, durable plastic pockets, etc.
- You have to like it: if green is your least favourite colour, don't have a green portfolio. It won't make a huge difference but if something is going to be around for a while it helps if you at least like the look of it.

You might keep your portfolio electronically. A nurse I know scans all his certificates and documents, keeps his reflections in Microsoft Word® documents, and stores them on a disk. He keeps a back-up and can print things down whenever he wants. The Royal College of Nursing 'Learning Zone' has an electronic portfolio for RCN members to use (http://www.rcn.org.uk, go to Learning Zone for more information).

Alternatively, you might want to use a 'ready-made' portfolio that guides you to include certain information. *The Churchill Livingstone professional portfolio* is a very useful PREP folder. I like it because it has a disk with documents you can print off, in addition to the documents already in the folder.

Whatever you choose, remember that PREP is not optional and that you shouldn't wait until the last minute. PREP is much more useful than simply proving your competence to the NMC (as if that alone weren't enough). It can also:

- help you with your appraisal
- help you fill out job applications
- help you get APEL (credit for prior experience and learning) for academic courses
- help you make out PDPs
- help you prove you have met KSF indicators.

The NMC handbook on PREP is an excellent document. It gives you extensive guidelines and information about how to manage your PREP. Just remember: your post-registration experience, education and practice belong to you, as an individual and a nurse.

PREP FAQs

Question: 'I've heard I can only put certificated, approved events into my PREP.'

Answer: 'No, you can put any experience into your portfolio as long as it shows your development as a nurse. The events don't need to be approved by anyone. Of course, the entire portfolio should show varied experiences, so there should be more than one type of experience or evidence.'

Question: 'After I re-register, I can bin all the old PREP stuff and start over, right?'

Answer: 'No, you should keep your old information, but you can move some of it to an archive file. It might be helpful later to have the information, and it could be very useful on reflection to look back and see how you have changed over the years as a nurse.'

Question: 'My employer asked me to show them my portfolio, but I heard they can't do that. Is that true?'

Answer: 'Yes, it's true. They can't ask to see your portfolio. It's yours; only the NMC can ask to see it. You can offer to show it to them, but it's up to you.'

Question: 'Is there a set format for the folder?'

Answer: 'No. It's up to you the way you arrange the folder, as long as you have all the information you need inside.'

Question: 'How do I know when I have had enough PREP?'

Answer: 'As a nurse, you probably never have enough informal learning, but there are two separate requirements for the renewal of your registration:

1. You have worked as a nurse/midwife for a minimum of 100 days (750 hours) in the past 5 years, or have taken an approved return-to-practice course.

2. You have recorded your continuing professional development over the 3-year registration period and can show that you have had at least 5 days (35 hours) of learning activities during the 3 years since your last registration.

   In addition, you must maintain a PPP and comply with any request from the NMC to audit your PPP/PREP.'

Question: 'Is PREP the same as my review at work?'

Answer: 'No, although you might put things you have learned at work into your PPP, PREP is about proving to the NMC that you have kept up to date.'

Question: 'Can I just print off my KSF outline to show I have met my PREP obligations?'

Answer: 'No, the NMC stipulates that you have to keep a portfolio.'

THE KNOWLEDGE AND SKILLS FRAMEWORK

Under Agenda for Change, each job must have a knowledge and skills framework (KSF). This has a number of purposes:

- to guide employees in the things they need to do to develop their role
- to outline the knowledge and skills needed to do a certain job
- to justify the need for training and development for an individual
- to give an outline for a review of performance
- to have fair and reasonable expectations for all employees.

It was developed so that it would be:

- easy to understand
- sensible
- applied across the NHS and across the UK
- a foundation for the skills and knowledge needed to deliver the services required
- about partnership between the NHS and those who work for the NHS.

The KSF has many different dimensions. Some of them will apply to everyone (core dimensions) and some will be a bit more specific. The core dimensions are:

- communication
- personal and people development
- health, safety and security
- service improvement
- quality
- equality and diversity.

The more specific dimensions are grouped into sections:

- health and well-being
- estates and facilities
- information and knowledge (information processing, collection and analysis)
- general (learning and development, development and innovation, finances, people management, etc.).

Each dimension is broken down into four levels, with indicators. The indicators discuss the way knowledge and skill should be applied at that level. For a person to be at a certain level, he or she needs to show he or she has met and can apply the knowledge and skill for that level. To make it easier, there are examples that illustrate how the KSF might be applied to different jobs.

The levels start with simple, personal expectations and end with complex expectations that impact across organisations. Think of them as concentric circles:

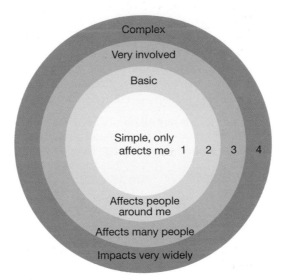

As an example, think of using a computer:

- Level 1: you would use your own computer to input and store information and data.
- Level 2: you would use your own computer to modify, structure and present data and information.
- Level 3: you would monitor the processing of data and information by other people.
- Level 4: you would develop and modify data and information management models and processes used by the whole organisation.

See? It goes from just worrying about yourself to working in a way that will influence many other people.

In the KSF, there are points called 'gateways'. To move past the pay point attached to that gateway, you and your manager will need to make a decision. There are two gateways in each band:

1. The foundation gateway: about 12 months after you start the job. This gateway asks you to have met all the basic, foundation knowledge and skill requirements for your post.
2. Second gateway: near the top of the band. This gateway asks you to show that you have met all of the knowledge and skill requirements to do your job.

You shouldn't have to worry too much about these gateways; you will discuss them with your manager as part of your review. It's a partnership: you and your manager should work together to make sure you are developing into your role as you should.

When you start your job, you should receive a copy of the KSF outline for that post, and you and your manager should sit down and agree how you will work to meet the expectations in the outline. Your manager has to help you by offering opportunities for training and education. It's your responsibility to take advantage of what is offered to you, and to speak up if you need more help.

The KSF has been developed to be fair, and to be easy to use. It's about there not being any surprises – you should know exactly what you are expected to know and to do. The Department of Health has excellent free publications about the KSF; these publications are available from the Department of Health website: http:www.dh.gov.uk

---

Summary

- It is your responsibility to keep track of your professional development.
- You have the right to be the kind of nurse you want to be, but to get there you have to plan ahead.
- You can use varied activities to meet your NMC requirement for continuous professional development.
- The KSF is there to help you identify what expectations there are for your level of knowledge and skill, and how your employer can help you learn and grow as a nurse.

11 Clinical governance

- Introduction
- Where does clinical governance come from?
- What is clinical governance?
- What does clinical governance mean to staff in the NHS?
- Organisations involved in clinical governance
- Summary
- Reference

INTRODUCTION

*I mean, this clinical governance stuff has nothing to do with me –
I'm just a staff nurse; I show up, I do as I am told and I go home.
Governance is something for the people in suits who tell people like
me what to do . . . (band 5 staff nurse)*

In this chapter, we will look at clinical governance, its impact on the
care nurses like you (and the nurse above) give every day and the
organisations that can give you information about clinical governance
and the issues it raises.

Although the principles of clinical governance apply across the
world, the different countries of the UK have different specific bodies
and policies involved in clinical governance. However, the basic information is applicable no matter where you live.

Just to make sure you understand the importance of clinical governance, I am going to try to put this to you in a different way:

Imagine that you have just bought a new car. You get home and
the key will not come out of the ignition. You ring the dealership
and speak to a secretary but she won't help you because she
doesn't sell cars herself. She puts you through to the person who
sold you the car but he says it's not his problem because he is
not a mechanic. You write to the people who made the car and
they say it's not their problem because they didn't put the key in
the ignition, you did. Everywhere you turn someone says it's
somebody else's problem: but all you want is a car that works,
that's what you paid for and that's what you need.

Wouldn't it have been helpful if the secretary had taken your name and address and sent someone out immediately to fix the car? Wouldn't you have expected the salesman to take responsibility for something he sold you? It was not either one of those individuals' fault that the key was stuck, but you relied on them and you needed them to help you.

How is it different from the care you give as a nurse under the NHS? You might not be the person who made the problem or who can fix the problem, in fact you might not know anything about the problem at all, but none of those things change the fact that the patient needs help and to the patient *you* are at the NHS.

Your nursing profession is like a treasure: it's a piece of property, it is something very valuable, and it's something you could potentially lose if you don't take care of it. Whenever you go to work you should be thinking about how well you are taking care of this treasure. Even if you don't care about your patients, even if you don't care about the hospital or organisation you work for, you *must* at least care about yourself: you need to prove you have maintained the skill and knowledge to work as a nurse, and then to use that skill and knowledge appropriately on every shift you work. If you fail to do these things, then get used to asking 'do you want fries with that?' because you are going to be serving burgers instead of doing medication rounds. Is that what you want?

You have to tell someone if you are not maintaining that standard so that they can help you, because if you don't, and something bad happens, you could wind up not only losing your profession but going to jail as well. If a patient is seriously injured or dies because you didn't keep up to date, then you are to blame.

You also have to tell someone if the organisation you work for is not doing things the way it should, because if you know but don't say anything, you are just as guilty as the rest of the organisation.

Clinical governance is making sure that the right people do the right things in the right way, every time.

WHERE DOES CLINICAL GOVERNANCE COME FROM?

Shortly after the general election in 1997, the Department of Health published *The new NHS, modern and dependable*, which promised that the NHS was to be reborn as an organisation with quality, professionalism and high standards at its core. Partly, this was in response to a number of stories in the media that exposed serious problems within the NHS, partly because – in the years leading up to the election – the NHS as an organisation hadn't seemed very trustworthy. Mistakes were made but instead of facing them openly, they were hidden and people suffered. Poorly performing professionals were shuffled around, and their lack of skills and their competence were never addressed. Leadership wasn't by clinicians but by business-people, who were more concerned about money than care, which meant that care often suffered.

It wasn't this way everywhere though: in some places the care was excellent and waiting times were very low; in other places, well, things were bad. Why were the good places so good? Why were the bad places so bad? Why couldn't the NHS deliver to the same standard across the entire nation?

In *The new NHS, modern and dependable*, the incoming government recognised that people wanted the highest level of care to be available where *they* lived, and began the discussion about how the NHS could be made to focus on patients and on patient care: clinical governance was chosen as the way forward. People wanted clinicians – not business-people – to make decisions about the best equipment, the best types of care and the right kinds of medication. The concept of clinical governance was new and fresh. It didn't involve blaming anyone but instead examined existing problems to see how things could be made better for patients, how care could be improved and how the number of people being cared for by the NHS could be increased.

In 1998, the Department of Health published *A first class service: quality in the new NHS*. This looked at the way care was delivered, the reason it was taking so long and promised to give England a first-class NHS, led by skilled clinicians who could offer the best standards of care.

WHAT IS CLINICAL GOVERNANCE?

A summary of *A first class service: quality in the new NHS* (Scally and Donaldson 1998) makes the following points about clinical governance:

- Clinical governance is the way by which the quality of care and capacity to deliver services, for the NHS in England, will reach and maintain high standards.
- Poor professional performance must be addressed and dealt with.
- Organisations must transform into ones with clinical leadership and positive cultures focused on what is best for patient care.
- Dealing with poor professional performance must be managed locally.

- The NHS has to learn from its past mistakes, through a system that allows news about good lessons to be shared, as well as mistakes and failures.

These really are the basics of clinical governance. Scally and Donaldson (1998) also give a definition of clinical governance:

> *A framework through which NHS organisations are accountable for continuously improving the quality of their services and safeguarding high standards of care by creating an environment in which excellence in clinical care will flourish.*

WHAT DOES CLINICAL GOVERNANCE MEAN TO STAFF IN THE NHS?

If you work in the NHS, you have an obligation to look at yourself the way the NHS looks at itself: you should look at the quality of the care you deliver, be willing to reflect on your actions and learn from your mistakes, as well as to learn what you do well. You need to both strive for excellence in care and make it possible for others to do the same.

The organisation you work for has a stake in making sure you offer the best nursing care possible: it will have to answer for mistakes you have made. It will be asked: 'Did anyone assess that nurse for competency? Was there anyone available to help that nurse do the right things?'. Your organisation must prove that yes, it assesses you, provides you with training and monitors your skills and abilities. This is done through your yearly performance review, through regular trainings and through any updates your employer might offer.

Even if you don't work in the NHS, you will probably be held to the same standard as a person in the same profession and at the same level in an NHS organisation. The level of professional behaviour and skill expected would be the same for a nurse whether she worked for the NHS or a private company.

One good thing about clinical governance is that it means that, if you *do* make a mistake, as long as you notify someone immediately, ask for help and can show that you did the best you could based on the information and resources you had available, you can't simply be blamed and fired. The organisation has to take more responsibility than ever to prove it supported you. People shouldn't feel bad about making mistakes if they are made honestly, but they shouldn't try to hide them or blame them on someone else.

ORGANISATIONS INVOLVED IN CLINICAL GOVERNANCE

Every NHS Trust has committees and groups that address the clinical governance needs of the organisation. For the remainder of this section I will simply call these 'clinical governance groups'.

These clinical governance groups will vary: some of them will receive material from the outside and determine if it is relevant to what is going on inside the organisation; some will look at this information to see how it compares with any goals the organisation might have been set; some will receive notification of complaints, accidents and incidents; some will look at clinical practice; some will look at human resources; some will look at training and education; some will look at leadership; some might look at communication. Or there might be one big group that does all of these things. It is not important how many groups there are; what is important is that the organisation does all of these things and can prove that it has done all of these things.

This is where you come in: you might be asked to be on one of these groups, although you are more likely to be asked to give feedback to one of them; you might be involved in a clinical audit; you might be asked to complete a staff survey; or you might be interviewed to discuss a serious incident or accident. All of these activities support clinical governance.

Many different models support clinical governance: at your level it is unlikely that you'll need to understand these in-depth models, although if you undertake further education it might be covered. What's important is that you understand that clinical governance is important to every person and at every level: patient to professional, HCA to medical consultant, domestic, trained nurse or director of human resources. In each of the models, clinical governance is represented as an ongoing cycle where information is gathered through audit and research, both inside and outside the organisation, is analysed and evaluated against benchmarks (standardised goals) and, as a result of that analysis, previous plans are evaluated and new plans are made, only to again go through the process of analysis and evaluation. Clinical governance is never-ending. As soon as you are sure you are doing the right thing, something's going to change.

But so far, that is looking at your own organisation. Outside of your organisation there are many other organisations that support clinical governance.

The Clinical Governance Support Team

By the time you read this, the Clinical Governance Support Team (http://www.cgsupport.nhs.uk) might not exist. As part of the ritual of reorganisation in the NHS, it is currently under review. However, at the time of writing, the Clinical Governance Support Team is responsible for putting out information, guidance and educational materials about clinical governance. The website contains numerous examples of best practice through the use of 'Eurekas' and other vignettes. Even if the team has ceased to exist, a search for clinical governance and 'Eurekas' might take you to this information. I sincerely hope that the review results in the continuation of this important organisation.

National Institute for Health and Clinical Excellence

The National Institute for Health and Clinical Excellence (NICE: http://www.nice.org.uk) sends out clinical guidance, technology appraisals, interventional procedures (what to do for certain types of problem) and public health advice. The extent to which each of these is applicable in the different countries of the UK varies, but no matter where you live they are good information; the only thing that changes is the applicability of the recommendation NICE makes. The website is an excellent source of information.

NICE is a quango: a quasi-autonomous non-governmental organisation. This means that although it sends out guidance on behalf of the government, it is not run by the government and is independent from the Department of Health (although some cynics say that it is impossible for anything that receives funding to be truly independent). There are a number of quangos: all it really means is they are not official governmental bodies.

The Healthcare Commission

The Healthcare Commission (http://healthcarecommission.org.uk) is another quango. Its role is to be the watchdog for the NHS – to ensure that quality is core to everything that is done, and that when things go wrong they are remedied. It is the role of the Healthcare Commission to monitor standards in areas such as cleanliness, waiting times and health and safety as part of a statutory duty to monitor the performance of NHS organisations in England.

The Healthcare Commission also responds to complaints that have been sent to different NHS organisations: if a patient or a family member complains to the Trust and are not happy with the response, they can involve the Healthcare Commission to make certain that all of the issues raised in the complaint have been addressed fully.

This is also the organisation that gives out 'star ratings' based on statistics, complaints and other key indicators of performance.

Summary

- Different organisations are involved in clinical governance: some give specific advice about governance; others provide guidance about practical issues.
- Everyone working in the NHS has a responsibility for clinical governance, both for themselves and for the organisation in which they work.
- NICE gives advice about different procedures, equipment, medication and technology. Although it is not applicable to every UK country, it still has good information.
- The Healthcare Commission monitors and assesses the NHS, making sure that complaints are followed up and that the organisation is meeting the targets and performance indicators it has been given.
- Each individual has to care about their practice, if for no other reason than if they don't, they will not be able to continue in practice.
- Reflection is a key component of your own personal clinical governance because it is the means by which you make sure that you are doing the right things, for the right reasons, in the right ways.

Reference

Scally G, Donaldson L 1998 The new NHS, modern and dependable (1997); A first class service: quality in the new NHS (1998). "Looking forward". British Medical Journal 317 61–65.

Index